Rosie's frank, informative and at times humorous account of a time in her life challenges so many preconceived ideas and thoughts on a cancer diagnosis. Her account of this part of her life journey is brutally honest which is refreshingly different from other related personal journals; instead of self-pity, sorrow and sadness, Rosie's book is inspiring and uplifting. Using NLP techniques she shows the reader how they can use their resources to create their own support which will be useful in any challenging situation not just going through a cancer diagnosis. Her positivity shines as brightly in this book as she does in life.

I very much hope that readers, whether the person diagnosed, their partner, a family member or friend, will have the opportunity to read Rosie's resourceful words and that it helps them to develop an understanding of how language and new ideas can lead to positive results.

Fiona JD Pearson, Friends of ANCHOR,
www.friendsofanchor.org

I think the main thing I should say about this book is it wasn't what I expected at all. I didn't expect to laugh more than I cried when reading this wonderful book. I've never read anything as positive or with so much courage about this subject, ever. I would recommend everyone should read this book, as we all will know someone whose life is 'interrupted' by cancer at some point. The advice given and the experiences shared have certainly opened my eyes to how I've already reacted when friends and family have faced such an interruption. The 'Top Top Tip' and 'Things I wish I'd known' list should be on the wall of every waiting room of every clinic across the country. I'm going to be a 'Positive Person' instead of a 'Negative Nelly' more often! And for the record, I'm from Middlesborough and yes I know what a bingo dress is ☺ Well done Rosie, a truly inspiring and 'different' book.

Marsha Dolan, Durham

Rosie's personal dialogue about her experience with breast cancer is frank and honest. Her open approach to a challenging and sometimes 'taboo' subject is both refreshing and empowering. She is passionate about conveying the importance of developing and maintaining a positive attitude, and she details how she used NLP techniques so that others may feel encouraged to model her approach. Rosie shows determination throughout, and this is more than matched by her 'wicked' sense of humour – I still giggle at the thought of Rosie imagining life with a false leg tucked in her bra – her idea of a prosthesis! It is a testament to Rosie's courage and generous nature that she has chosen to share her thoughts and feelings through *No More Bingo Dresses*, and I am sure this will empower others facing a similar journey.

Karen Moxom, Managing Director, The Association for NLP (ANLP), www.anlp.org

Step into the mind of Rosie O'Hara and feel the positive vibe! In the last year I have encountered a few 'bumps in my road' which I had a hard time dealing with. Without me knowing it I used a 'model' similar to NLP to cope with what was presented and to get myself off that feeling-sorry-for-myself-spot. Little did I realise that I was missing out on one thing: negative words are banned.

This book is a page turner. It leads you through Rosie's world filled with humour (very dark humour at times but with that ever sparkling shine of a Compelling Purpose) and enjoying whatever comes your way following a system which uses words and language to be positive and to be in a good and useful state. This book is touching and entertaining and I'm very sure that every reader that is open to new ideas (or ideas already known but learning is a life-long process) will thoroughly enjoy Rosie's style and wit.

Little did Rosie know that when she asked me to read this book she not only gave me the great honour of reading it before print but she also gave me the precious gift of learning about NLP and how NLP can help me and everybody else to grow and develop positively. Rosie, thank you very much for changing my Map of the World.

Daniel Ketelaar, Kinloss

Of Rosie's previous book a reviewer commented, was 'like sitting down with a friend over a cup of coffee'. The same is true of *No More Bingo Dresses*; it is chatty, intimate, and like most conversations, it doesn't go in a straight line. NLP was clearly an enormous help in managing her disease in a planned and positive way; elements of the theory are interwoven with a very honest account of day to day experiences and feelings. I think many will enjoy sharing this particular cup of coffee with Rosie.

Alastair Cunningham, Scottish Clans and Castles Ltd

Rosie has a delightful unassuming style. This book is written in a blog format which is refreshingly direct. As you might expect from a serious NLP professional, there is some subtlety but no mumbo-jumbo.

Many people will gravitate toward the action plan; however there is power on each page delivered in a simple and honest fashion. How Rosie beat cancer and is medication free is both humorous and inspiring.

George McBride, Coaching For Teachers Academy

No More Bingo Dresses is not a page-turner, and thank goodness for that. This story could be told by millions, but each 'page' would be different because cancer is like that. Rosie tells it like it is, the mood swings, terror to boredom to being able to share with others. I am better for having read Rosie's story.

Edward P Gibson, FBI (retired) 1985-2005

No More Bingo Dresses

Rosie O'Hara

ISBN Paperback 9781908218346, ISBN ePub 9781908218360, ISBN Mobipocket 9781908218353.

Published in the UK by MX Publishing, 335, Princess Park Manor, Royal Drive, London, N11 3GX

www.mxpublishing.co.uk

Cover design by www.staunch.com

I dedicate this book to Jim Symon, with whom so many things are possible, Rebecca (not her name but she chose to remove herself from my life after having been a steadfast friend – such is life), my daughter Kristin Rietsch, and my grandsons Leon and Nico, the source of so much joy, and in no particular order, Alasdair Gordon, David Taylor, Sara Hunt (the Pilates whiz), Caitlin Collins (who helped me increase my awareness of my use of NLP), Ian Parfitt (who encouraged me to go snorkelling in the Red Sea), my son Jacob O'Hara, Gina Pickersgill (who picked me up on my language in November 2009 – well done that woman and thanks for your support), everyone of my Facebook friends up to and including 26th February 2009 who supported me with many good words, those on my NLP Practitioner Course in Aberdeen in the 'Class of 2009', in particular Susan Raeper, and all those mentioned in this book who sent me kind words and good thoughts too. And my Mum and Dad, Maureen and Ron Savage, who started my journey in life for me (and I suspect had they known how 'interesting' some of it might be, they might have changed their minds ☺)

Acknowledgements

My thanks go to Robert A Eslinger, DO, HMD, and owner of Reno Integrative Medical Center, Reno, Nevada for his permission to use the work of Dr Brodie who died in 2005.

And my thanks go to Shelle Rose Charvet for her permission to use her article 'Ten Top Tips to Survive the Healthcare System', as well as her work using the LAB (Language and Behaviour) Profile and her book *Words That Change Minds*, which in part helps me just to survive most days ☺

In respect of the lyrics to 'Someone to Watch Over Me', the copyright on Gershwin's lyrics expired in 2007 in the European Union, where this book originates.

My acknowledgments go to everyone in the world of NLP whose books and articles I have read, trained with, been trained by and those who attended my training courses and workshops/presentations especially in the period from 26th January 2009 to the beginning of May 2009. You inspire me too ☺

Foreword

As a full-time Hospice Counsellor of several years and an NLP Practitioner, I am absolutely delighted to introduce such an inspiring book. The experience of cancer can be, for many people, a powerless journey into a black abyss. Read on, and Rosie will show you how it can be, so very different. Rosie writes with humour – which is therapeutic in itself – and with honesty, courage and an openness into her world which is breathtakingly refreshing. She uses all the internal resources that she can muster and readily draws on her vast knowledge of NLP and uses these elements as if soldiers in a focussed and determined army, with her in command.

And, believe me, as I've witnessed for years, a person can and does influence their own personal journey for good or otherwise. I use NLP in my practice and I've seen transformations in people in a matter of minutes – completely changing how they experience their challenge on their journey. People can choose to live with optimism, in the moment, with their focus on a positive future, however they perceive that to be. Hats off to Rosie. This book will empower and bring hope to those encountering a challenge, and to others who may need a nudge to realise that human potential is powerful vast.

Julia Sixsmith, Hospice Counsellor and NLP Practitioner,
Wigan & Leigh Hospice

Preface

Originally called 'My Left Breast', *No More Bingo Dresses* started out life as a way of letting friends and family know that I had discovered I had 'a little breast cancer', as my 'breast care' nurse informed me, and a way of keeping sane, in particular in the time between 26th January and 26th February 2009, and later as well, believe me. Along the way I collected information and comments from friends: 'you should share this you know', 'other women (well in my world this applied to anyone male or female) need to know', 'we don't talk enough about this'. And do you know what? I started to agree with these comments, that generally we hear about the bad stuff, the people who died, the people who 'fought' and 'battled against' and 'overcame' cancer. I think it's a dis-ease and my body was not at ease, and more on that later. I had another major op over 30 years ago that was also serious and no one said any of those things about that. I think we are scared of the word cancer and quite rightly so and I think because of that we go into 'freeze frame', 'rabbit in the headlights mode' and we don't act as usefully as we might do. I also noticed over the past year (as this is now September 2010) that many women adopt an attitude of 'putting it behind them', more in a way of forgetting (because it's that thing that you don't really want to talk about, do you?).

So this is 'my take' on my breast cancer and, as my breast care nurse at one point pointed out to me, I am different to other women. Yes well, I've grown up knowing that and since 1994, I've also grown up a bit more and I know it's ok to be different and it's ok to be me, and being me I can actually help and apparently inspire others. So I hope that you find this entertaining (it is meant to be – some bits are very funny and oh! very real) and useful. Remember, I'm not and not claiming to be an expert on cancer or treatments, but I am a human being, I'm a Mum, I'm a Granny, I'm a partner to my man Jim, and I am somewhat an expert at using and training NLP (Neuro Linguistic Programming – stay with me, you'll find out more in this book) and I need, like we all do, 'a little help from my friends' (especially when we're out of tune).

Cancer is not an 'illness', you can't 'catch it', it's not something you 'deserve'. In fact there are so many unknowns in respect of cancer and how it develops and forms; it's a very complex area. The medical model looks for statistics, generalisations and hones in on those statistics and generalisations (more on those later) and, dependent on whom you are talking to at the time, they 'have the answer' and then low and behold someone else, somewhere else has a different answer.

Fact is, in terms of the language used around cancer and its treatment, there is an awful lot of negativity. I've had experience of cancer twice, once I was married to a man who died as a result of where his tumour was located and that's another story. And then in 2009 when I was going in one direction and lots of curious things were happening with the World Economy, I found I had a tumour in my left breast.

Every day I work with language, noticing its use and the effects it has on us. This book describes how I dealt with things (lots of things, and people and most important of all me) in respect of the cancer that I had and what was happening around me.

Believe me if for one second I had found it 'a struggle', a battle', 'difficult', 'hard', 'emotional turmoil', or anything else that trips lightly off the tongue, this book wouldn't be here. It wasn't something to overcome! I don't do hills. It was, oh no, another challenge, in my life! My biggest challenge was other people's words. I saw an obstacle and I chose to either get round this obstacle, or build a tunnel through it, or underneath it and get out the other side, and in so doing let the whole mass of heavy problem-making words disintegrate.

My plea to everyone, see the Individual (the person), not the word Cancer, listen to what this individual person has to say, as an individual and find out how they personally feel and think and how they construct their world. Put anything and everything that you know and believe to be true on one side and listen to that individual, please.

Contents

Acknowledgements..vii

Foreword..ix

Preface x

Contents

27th January 2009: Good and useful state 1

Telling my friends...7

NLP stuff: This good and useful state 10

NLP stuff: Tips for good listening...................................14

NLP stuff: Presuppositions or Operating Beliefs of NLP....19

31st January 2009: So where do I begin? 21

1st February 2009: The castor oil story to brighten your day.....23

NLP stuff: Words...28

NLP stuff: Words and wheelbarrows...............................31

4th February 2009: Oh doctors 37

NLP stuff: State Maintenance and Second Positioning 41

1st February 2009: To detox or not to detox....................46

The cancer personality 48

NLP stuff: Creating a compelling purpose 55

12nd February 2009: My state maintenance slipped 58

NLP stuff: Dealing with an incident from the past............62

16th February 2009: Getting plastered 65

NLP stuff: Visualisation 71

17th February 2009: Aberdeen 74

18th February 2009: Aberdeen 76

19th February 2009: Aberdeen 78

21st February 2009: The conservatory diary extract 79

23 February 2009: My sister 86

I'm goin' to live forever...93

25th February 2009: Keeping you abreast of the situation........97

2nd March 2009: Not lobster pots then?..........................103

3rd March 2009: Reshaping my life 105

8th March 2009: Softees 113
11th March 2009: This convalescing lark.....................118
My compelling purpose 124
Exercising or regaining movement! 126
23rd April 2009: This prosthesis thing, breast form, chicken
fillet! 131
Thoughts and experiences with breast forms...............134
The Red Sea..136
Oh hell – other people – it's me who had the cancer! 139
Employment Support Allowance..................................142
'When my granny had two boobs!' 145
NLP stuff: It's fine to be a 'Positive Person' or a 'Negative
Nelly' 147
NLP stuff: Submodalities..154
Time to decide 158
NLP stuff: A possible way to plan..............................163
NLP stuff: Ten Top Tips to Survive the Healthcare System 166
Things I wish I'd known..170
Other women's stories 171
NLP stuff: On getting other people to 'go with you'................185
And I almost forgot to say 188
Out of alignment 190
Bibliography 192
Glossary of NLP terminology.....................................193

This book is not a replacement for any medical, mental or physical issues that need attention by a relevant professional. All readers are urged to seek proper professional medical and psychological advice as appropriate.

27th January 2009: Good and useful state

I can't go swimming this morning cos someone's punctured my left water wing. My friend Rebecca is going to the hospital with me on Friday to find out 'what happens next?' – more laughter please (cos I know she has a wicked sense of humour).

Mmm, well, 'a good and useful state' is one of my favourite sayings and doings.

On Monday 26th January, I went for a core biopsy and let me tell you it was sore – okay maybe it is just the pressure – but the pressure of a small baby elephant several times, and one of the times was sore. I was busy throughout all this, singing 'I'm gonna live forever' – Irene Cara in *Fame* (in my head) – I'm going to live forever, well at least to 97. The nurse was asking me if I was okay – I had to stop her and tell her she was interrupting my singing and I would let her know if I wasn't okay.

My daughter (Kristin) who likes gory stuff (or she's just plain inquisitive) and is 32 (well 2 days off being 33) was with me. We were laughing and cracking jokes, in the 'core biopsy room' – no idea what its real name is. The doctor carrying out the procedure joined in, the other one was a bit serious and she looked a bit malnourished, perhaps she needed some chicken soup (Kristin said). Where do these people come from?

The breast care nurse (I'd quite like her to care for me not just my breast) was a tad on the serious side too, seemed disappointed that I wasn't going to cry when she told me it wasn't a cyst like my Mum had at my age (damn), but a 'little breast cancer'. My friend Rebecca asked later is that like 'a little bit pregnant'. Kristin did say that on the scan the tumour looked like an embryo and she was expecting to hear how many months the baby was (I had my eyes closed).

Later that day I was shattered and feeling sick – too many Thornton's Continental Chocolates do not make you feel good, on the contrary ☹

So I didn't want any tea. Later I asked Jim would he please go to the shop and get me a baguette. Did you know a baguette is a word that can be so misunderstood [in NLP terms it's a generalisation, as baguette covers many things] and did you know this misunderstanding could have dire consequences? Relationships can break down as a result of misunderstandings like the one that followed. 'You're not listening to me, you don't care . . .', that kind of thing.

I suggested Jim go in the Co-op and ask for a baguette (when in doubt ask the staff – what are they there for?) and that a part-baked baguette was okay. Jim returned a whole while later and thrust (nicely) two cheese and garlic baguettes (from Tesco, I don't shop there) under my nose (bear the chocolates in mind here). Now for me cheese and garlic is not a good combination (and certainly not after chocolate), so I said in a small voice 'I don't think I fancy that'. 'Well that's the kind of baguette we had the other day' he retorted somewhat irritated – yes loosely I would agree. We had had spaghetti at the weekend and with the spaghetti, garlic bread (baguette). But I wanted a baguette that was crunchy and untainted by garlic that I could put butter and jam on and I was close to tears.

Then from out of nowhere a major crisis erupted – suddenly 'I always tell Jim he is wrong', 'I always tell him he goes the wrong way, does the wrong thing'.

Somehow, my head felt all of this was unjust. So I got up off the couch and followed him into the kitchen. And through my tears of frustration at the baguette (and him perhaps) and my tears of anger at the 'little breast cancer' (I can't schedule this in my diary and I realise I may have to – this might have to become 'Scheduling this in my diary will be a really good idea and I want to make time for this'). I held onto the kitchen island (as in cupboard, not that we have big pieces of land floating around the kitchen). Breathed deeply through all this mess and thought of a good and useful state and explained:

'My name is not Helen [his previous wives were both called Helen, second wife died of breast cancer, first wife of bowel cancer], this is my breast cancer and this is me. Please, I don't know if you are confusing me with something from your past. That's bad for me and you if it's something that happened in the past that was with someone else. I don't want this breast cancer; I want to live (''light up the sky with my name'') forever. I have lots to do (places to go, people to see, I want to be there for my grandsons, for my children, I want to buy a new motorbike, I want to enable more people to do what they want to do!)' I continued, 'if you want me to, I can go with my ''little breast cancer'' to Aberdeen [we rented a flat there for work], and live in the flat there. From there I could manage to walk to the Spar shop and get a baguette and no one would argue with me. I can manage to look after myself. This was not in my life plan.'

I think I said some other things. What was important about these things for our relationship, for the whole cancer stuff and for my life and our life together and everything else that is still happening, is that I thought about the kind of words that Jim understands. I thought about the kind of things that he does and I spoke to him in his words, so I used phrases like he uses (the ones that sometimes 'drive me up the wall'). I kept away from accusations, anger, tears, 'you make me', 'you never' phrases, etc. Because somewhere deep down inside I was starting to create a plan. Well actually it's a Compelling Purpose, in my jargon, that's 'a plan' to other people, and I started to think about how I was/we were going to cope with this change and how to get what was right for me, and what was right for us and right out in the future are stood two wee boys growing up, and their mum (Kristin) and their uncle (Jacob) and me and Jim, and lots of other people I will somehow touch, inspire (I find this very odd, me inspire people?), or whatever and all of this is at this point in time very faint, but it's there.[1]

Then Jim decided to cheer up a bit, we had a hug and he decided he would sort himself out and get fit to deal with all this with me.

Well thank goodness, I'm not really fussed on doing this by myself, like so many things beforehand in my life.

I find it's easier to tell some people face to face, but with some it's not possible and some I wanted to know pdq for support. For them I've started an irregular email diary [this backfired a

---

[1] I only became aware of all of what I had created at this point in time (this 'coping in a crisis') 7 weeks after my op, when I was interviewed by Caitlin Collins, a reporter for the ANLP (Association of Neuro Linguistic Programming) magazine *Rapport*. She asked me a question and suddenly I remembered, this is an innate skill I have, it was modelled from me in 1995 by a man carrying out his Master Practitioner modelling. NLP is based on how people do things well and when we do something really well, there are two aspects: (1) we don't know we do it and (2) we don't know how we do it. Thanks to that chap Richard Royce, I do know that I can do it and how I do it and I use the skill more effectively, because years ago I would let things spiral into the depths of despair first. Thanks also to Cricket Kemp who recognised I could do it. And anyone can learn it – ask me how.

little later in respect of one person, but that backfiring helped me to help myself in another way – so there's no such thing as failure – only feedback, and feedback is there to be learned from], not sure that my Mum was too fussed about this email attachment thing, but oh at nearly 80 she does email all right (she was having a font problem I then discovered).

I tried to set up a lunch meet with my middle 'daughter-in-law' [strictly speaking 'step-daughter' but I hate the 'step' bit], she's the closest geographically – but she wanted to know why beforehand and then she cried on the phone – this is not good, I was hoping to avoid that. We still met for lunch and it was good (only taken 2 years to arrange this, but there were other things that got in the way before).

Telling my friends

I'm writing this and sending it to you in the first place, as you are someone I'd like to share this with (lucky you, you might think when you read what it says later).

Now, firstly I am not out for the sympathy vote, secondly I'd like some support from you, as someone I know, value and trust as being a supportive person and (I hope) understanding and appreciating my humour. It will be rather black at times, Gallows Humour.

By the way, 'sorry' is banned – it's banned in my life unless you can really justify using it, so no 'sorry to hear that' – this is a learning curve for us all. No 'I had a friend who . . .'

Last week I met lots of people who told me how inspiring I am (I remembered I appreciate better what people have to say about me when I see it written down. So I wrote lots of notes in my head and looked at them – those of you not much acquainted with NLP are on a learning curve here ☺). [We'll come to what NLP is soon, but some people like to see things, notes, cards, flowers etc., some people like people to say good things about them (has a slight downside that as we more often concentrate on the negative), and other people like to do things with other people or have them done for them to know that they have been appreciated.]

Yesterday I discovered I have 'a little breast cancer' (please note in terms of NLP – Deletions, Distortions and Generalisations – this means I don't know enough from this statement about what the diagnosis means – should I worry, how much should I worry and all manner of things there is just insufficient information). Now I know what 'a little night music' is, but what is this?

I need your support please (my first stop is my bra of course – ah shopping). What does that mean? Lots of laughter, and please – sideways glances, whispering behind my back, feeling sorry for me (or yourself) [I discovered that one later] are all no nos. (And if I get stroppy or more stupid than ever – please tell me, this is really not an excuse).

I'm sore and annoyed (at me primarily – how dare this happen?). I need to reorganise this 'breast care' stuff – support nurse rapport at that point in time scored 0 out of 10 [more on this 'rapport' and why it's so important later], listening and questioning of patient as an individual varies from 9 to about 2. And polar bears (a threatened and dying out species) on the ceiling of the 'examination room' well I ask you. Wait 'til I get to fill out the feedback form!

Fortunately I had Kristin (daughter) with me and my 'tit-ex', some of that stuff you use to white out mistakes you've made when you've written something, in my handbag as it happens.

You know, Tip-Ex. Kristin found it when she was searching for a hairbrush. She wondered if it would work on the tumour, it didn't ☺ the little breast cancer is still there.

NLP stuff: This good and useful state

Perhaps first, it would help if I explained a little about this NLP. NLP stands for Neuro Linguistic Programming: Neuro refers to the brain and nervous system, Linguistic is the verbal and non-verbal language used to communicate, and Programming is the unique way you put it all together to create behaviour.In a nutshell (and there is so much more to it than this):

NLP started out in the Human Potential Movement, which started in Esalen, a small community at Big Sur near Santa Cruz, Southern California in the 1970s. The key leaders of the Human Potential Movement were Fritz Perls (Gestalt therapy), who was the first resident scholar in Esalen, Gregory Bateson (philanthropist, anthropologist, systems thinker amongst other things, who is credited with having brought together John Grinder and Richard Bandler, who today are often credited with 'starting NLP'), who was the last resident scholar in Esalen, and Virginia Satir, who was last in charge of training at Esalen (Virginia's work is fundamental to the NLP Meta Model on these Distortions, Deletions and Generalisations, which are minefields in communication).

The Human Potential Movement is the source of the NLP presuppositions (more later on the NLP presuppositions that make understanding other people and ourselves easier). The psychology of the Human Potential Movement is about how people grow and develop positively – the bright side of human nature. Abraham Maslow was the first to model successful people in the 1940s in terms of 'pushing the farthest reaches of human nature'. Maslow's work created the new positive psychology of generative change, rather than remedial change.

NLP is a communication model about human behaviours, and using it successfully we can 'run our own brain' (and that means our emotions or feelings as they are often called) and create more resourcefulness, and access, and put into practice our highest potentials and possibilities.

If that was a bit much for you or a bit too highbrow, can you just accept it's great, it works, for anyone who wants it to work for them? Just bear with me, and I promise I'll give you more and more examples of how it works and you can apply it too. (Not just for cancer; it works for many things.)

Now one of the main things when we (my Associates and I) start to enable people to do things (or train) using NLP, is that either as a Practitioner of NLP or for you to do something, anything, it's really important to be in a good and useful state. Not any old state, a good and useful one.

So how did I do this? When I was told it's a 'little breast cancer', momentarily I went into denial (not that river in Egypt ☺) and I noticed a dark cloud begin to descend around me and down and around me, and I noticed 'my nose is still peeking out' (a bit like over the duvet or blanket. So immediately what I did was think and it was very, very rapid: 'I have two grandsons Leon (5) and Nico (almost 3), and I love them to bits and I want to be there for them, present in person.' 'I want to be there for their Mum, cos she has no Dad any more, and it's her birthday on Wednesday and we're going out for tea', and 'hell I've got a business to run and people to enable using NLP and it's only January and I had other plans, seriously.'

Next I breathed, and my head started coming up out of the dark cloud, and the dark cloud was disappearing and I started to see more clearly, and pressure (that I hadn't noticed before) lifted from chest. I relaxed back into the chair I was sat in and felt the chair supporting me and 'I started to make a plan'. That's a favourite saying of mine, and it means I start to make a plan, there needs to be silence around me, and in my head, and I start to plan. Or in this case I started to be open to a plan, because I HAVE NOT DONE THIS BEFORE, ME, HAVE CANCER, ME, IT DOESN'T HAPPEN TO ME! I NEED A PLAN (aka a Compelling Purpose.)

What happens next is I think of all the things that won't happen if I'm not there, I think of the commitments I have, where's my diary. I think 'oh shit' and the plan starts.

Step 1: What does this mean?

Step 2: Listen carefully

Step 3: Weigh up all the options

And there will be more steps. I haven't met them yet.

I also notice I am relaxing; I have arms and legs uncrossed.

I can start to face the world. There will be more on good and useful states later.

NLP stuff: Tips for good listening

These tips are good for you to listen to anyone – if you have cancer these tips will be useful to enable you to understand more about what people (friends, employers, healthcare professionals etc.) are saying and then later to question what the other people say (and think about how you say things in a more useful way – more on this in Words and wheelbarrows later as well).

Focus and put your attention on what the other person is actually saying, rather than on the other person and what you think is the right way.

Give the other person time. Wait for your chance to talk. Allowing them space to share their problems helps you and the other person to understand more clearly what the problem is for the other person.

Mentally create your own picture (or whatever other way you remember things that have been said) of what the other person is saying, but remember it is just your own picture, not theirs.

Repeat back **exactly what the other person says, in the other person's words or phrases, exactly as the other person said them**. This helps the other person to know that you are really listening, and it saves you trying to understand the other person by 'interpreting' what they say.

You know that voice in your head (we all have one)? Turn it down or off (it's possible, honest). Having a real interest in what the other person is saying helps us concentrate better on the other person.

Pay close attention to the words that the other person is emphasising and repeating (listen out for repeated words and phrases; they sometimes emphasise something in their tone, or the way they use their hands or look in a particular direction).

Ask yourself if the other person has finished thinking. Do their eyes look like they're still considering what they've just said? (People move their eyes when they are thinking!)

Soft focus your eyes in order to take in the whole scene rather than looking into other person's eyes. There's so much going on in a conversation you'll miss things that are going on if you insist on looking in their eyes. This can help put things in perspective. You'll also notice their gestures more; remember their gestures are just their gestures, avoid reading something into the gestures.

Rapport

So when my support nurse leant into me with her legs crossed and leaning on one elbow, it was like the world's worst invasion of my private space. (Kristin commented had my support nurse sneezed, my head would have been through the back of the sofa I was sat on!) It's really important at any time when you're conversing with another person, especially when you want to give someone bad information, when you want to show someone you are really listening, that you match or mirror their body posture. So she should have sat back and copied what I was doing. At that precise moment in time I hated her, she was in my space, taking my breath away, interfering with my thoughts and when she asked me if I understood, yes I did and it would have been better for me if she had sat back.

For some reason, some schools of thought believe that you 'should' lean in towards the other person: no, no, no. Match or mirror what they are doing – people like people who are like themselves. When you approach a person, whether sitting or standing, notice how they are sitting or standing and gently and unobtrusively start to match or mirror the other person's posture. Not straight away, and it doesn't have to be exact, particularly if the person you are matching has a physical limitation. If they shift their position you may have to drift across to the new position over time. This will help you understand the other person better, yes really.

Now there are might be problems, if you are very much taller than the other person, or the other person is much taller than you, or there is a great weight difference. What to do? Well if you are tall – get your eyes at roughly their level, so sit on the edge of a table or suggest you both sit down (my granny was a very short lady and she used to complain that at business dinners with my grandfather she had to get a chair to stand on to speak to most people – not sure if this is a true fact!).

Try approximately copying (this is far more subtle than mimicking) the other person's gestures, especially if you tend to sit still. For someone who moves about a great deal, people who sit still are often perceived as not listening to the other person. The more you practise, breathing becomes identical, skin tone starts to match, you move your head at the same time, you may find yourself even scratching just after they have done this (be careful here ☺). Watch people in bars and coffee shops, or people who are just getting on well.

You can notice breathing by the rise and fall of people's shoulders (a safe place to look, believe me, especially if you are a man!).

Never copy any gesture you are uncomfortable with; the other person will notice.

Your physical movement and behaviour will really affect your ability to get into rapport and people will listen to you much more openly and know they are being listened to!

Occasionally it's handy, when you have got good rapport to slightly change things. Think it about it, if the person you are speaking to is upset and finding it difficult to change that or if they are having difficulty 'seeing the wood for the trees', then you might want to make use of the good rapport and sit back yourself, gently. Thus leading them to sit back or ask them to get up and 'have a think about things in a different way'. It's amazing what shifting our position will do for us in terms of helping us to think more clearly.

NLP stuff: Presuppositions or Operating Beliefs of NLP

Presuppositions, or operating beliefs of NLP, These are the principles or suppositions on which NLP is based; remember NLP is purely a model with which to negotiate life better, so

I'm using 'presuppositions' in the 'No More Bingo Dresses' context.

People respond to their map of reality and not to reality itself. We all create our own reality, whatever reality is, made of sights, sounds and feelings, past experiences, beliefs and values to name but a few things. We all experience the world differently from one another: ask any five people you know what comes into their heads when you say the following words, separately: Elephant, Alarm, Velvet, Lemon and Smoke. People respond to their Model or Map of the World: a person's values, beliefs and attitudes, as well as their internal representations, states and physiology, which all relate to and create their belief system of how the world operates. This relates to Korzybski's General Semantics[2] and his discussion of our Map or Model of the World – the map is not the territory.

---

[2] www.gestalt.org/semantic.htm.

All behaviour has a positive intention. People are always trying to achieve something valuable for themselves and others although not always in your model of the world. What sometimes appeared as unuseful for me was only that way because it didn't fit in with my model; for the other person it was the right thing to do or say.

People make the best choice they can at the time. Knowing whatever the person did was the best choice they could make that fitted in with their map of the world helped me understand it was about them and not about me and I can either listen to their well-meaning advice or walk away.

We already have all the resources we need or we can create them. We can create resourceful states, for example for listening, for being in a good place when going for the op, or having needles inserted (I really dislike needles).

The mind and body are one system. Changing things in our body will affect our mind if we let that happen, conversely changing things in our mind (a good and useful state) will affect our body and our healing for example.

31st January 2009: So where do I begin?

Good job I went to the hospital at 1 p.m. yesterday (Friday) and not 4.30 p.m. on Wednesday (Kristin's birthday) as I would have had to go back again. We were there for hours.

My consultant is very pleasant (far too young for me to call him Mr), but for once I didn't argue ☺ and he has a sense of humour, the breast care nurse who we saw briefly before seems to have developed better rapport skills (perhaps she read a book on NLP during the week? ☺). My sterling support Rebecca was with me – ever heard that phrase, 'your friendship is priceless' – heavens, what that woman puts up with, with me!

You're not waiting for me to 'get on with it', are you?

Well there's good news and bad news, the good news is I'll be around for a long time yet. Mixed response to that I bet ☺

The bad news, well kind of, is that I'll be shape shifting, i.e. becoming rather flat on the left side. So I'm going to get a plaster cast done of the left boob and then I think a fetching bronze would be nice as a display object, perhaps not too heavy in case Nico lobs it somewhere, though knowing him, he and his brother will fight over it to take to bed. A comforting thought.

I'll find out the beginning of next week when the op is and someone mentioned it will take 6 weeks to convalesce – I'm sure they meant 6 days – it will be business as usual NLP-wise, no getting out of courses – for anyone apart from me, briefly perhaps.

This week has been a bit wearing in some ways – I do cry you know, but not a lot as it gives me a headache and it's so unuseful, can't be doing with other people crying. (Check out – is about you or your past? Then get a grip). Life goes on you know, we know it does in our family (whilst editing this chapter I heard Freddy Mercury on the radio – I know he's dead – singing 'The Show Must Go On' – indeed).

And by the way, I have thought about all this, I've looked at the possibilities and I've talked it through with the doctor and me and I've felt how I will feel about it (hey, weight loss, I know a bit drastic) and unusually for me I'll have to do some things that others tell me to do ☺

Off shopping for some new bras, a cookery book (from the Phoenix Store in Findhorn) and probably some healthy things.

Oh yes and when all this all over, who's for joining me in platform shoes and glittery stuff to sing 'Supertrooper' and 'Dancing Queen'?

1st February 2009: The castor oil story to brighten your day

Well I did some reading over the weekend and now have questions to ask of surgeon. I also contacted remaining two 'daughters-in-law'.

I went to Findhorn on Saturday morning, not, I hasten to add, for some spiritual healing, nor because I needed the vibes or whatever, but because I wanted a book and some organic stuff (does chocolate porridge count?). I bumped into a friend I haven't seen for over a year since she sold her shop in Nairn (curious, this re-finding people, been happening since last November, mmm . . .).

I purchased a very interesting, objective book which has given rise to the questions I will ask later today and the castor oil (which I went back to purchase on Sunday), along with a small statue of Tara the Hindu goddess (it spoke to me), and a crystal angel (if you are on Facebook, I'm collecting Guardian angels, please send me several). Tara incidentally is the Goddess of Compassion, One Who Saves, Diamonds are Her Sacred Stone. (I quite like that thought – I have Armani Diamonds – for the unknowing, it's a perfume). I particularly like this bit about Tara: she is the Mother of Liberation and represents the virtues of success in work and achievements and her name means 'star'.

We had Leon and Nico (my grandsons) from Saturday afternoon until yesterday before lunch. It was good fun. Jim was a great help as this time he put the beds up and put them down (this dis-ease has advantages – maybe the biggest one is letting me know I am not invincible and I really might stop this 'needing to do everything for everyone else'). Jim sent Leon up the loft to put some things up there – this is the equivalent of sending small boys up chimneys ☺ Leon thought it was great to be up there by himself and Jim thought it was great he could stay on the ground. Nico missed this, he was busy with Granny. Jim then took Leon off to move the bowls carpets, Leon had his first introduction to bowls – this is the way of getting young blood into the bowling club ☺ Nico and Granny ate healthy spelt biscuits ☺, along with fresh bread.

Tea was as every meal with small children – interesting – and bedtime was a different tussle as Leon had earache and Nico jumping on his head didn't help, but we got Leon to bed and let Nico wear his batteries out (when I find out where you insert them, I'll remove 'em earlier).

Breakfast on Sunday was for the guys a four-course affair, starting with healthy soya milk hot chocolate and soya and banana smoothie made by Granny and degenerating into nougat pillows and half a buttery when Jim got up ('Jim, we was starving waiting for you' – no prizes for guessing who said that).

Now back to the book, it tells me 'Amazon', as in women not the bookstore, means without a breast. The Amazon women had a breast removed to improve their aim with the long bow. So the author of the book asks 'do you want to improve your aim?' Well, what a silly question to ask me. But also I was always rubbish at archery so perhaps, you never know, improving my aim in life can only be good ☺

Now the book also suggests various remedies to try at home, one of which is a compress. The most easily available oil from the book was castor oil, so I bought some; interestingly it gets infused just round the corner from me in Tytler Street. Apparently you bake a cloth soaked in the oil in the oven and then wrap the baked cloth in other cloths or plastic (good job I left the plastic out, as I found out later). Now some of you will know at times I tend to abandon anything I am cooking, one of my readers of this diary will tell you 'I always thought carrots should be burnt as a child' – this was in my early caramelising experimental days ☺ So I abandoned the baking cloth to its baking and may have been in my Facebook account uploading photos. Eventually I realised 'I must take cloth out of oven'. It was smelling a little burned, but I duly wrapped it in two other cloths and applied them all to the lumpy part of my breast as I lay reclining on the sofa watching CSI Sunday. My eyes watered, largely due to the accompanying burning smell which I thought I had released from the oven. The cloths seemed to be getting hotter, so I took them into the utility room (this was about half an hour later), and oops as I put them in the sink to rinse them, I discovered they were slowly combusting away, as they burst into flames in the sink – ah, narrow escape there and rather drastic really – but burning the tumour out might have worked ☺

By the way, words like 'rough', 'tough', 'problem', 'difficult', 'illness', 'struggle', 'fight' etc. are banned – at some point there will be a short intermission until normal service (with a better aim) is resumed.

My favourite quotes of last week from my friends:

'I learned long ago that Rosie lives her life to the beat of her own drum! I'm singing with you!' Joanna Pirie, The Money Coach

'Amongst other things, Rosie, u taught me ways in which to regain my strength, self worth, resistance and passion for life! Your letter was admirable. I'm with you baby!' Liz McGhee – my latest Master Practitioner and woman I admire (31 years old and four children on her own ranging from toddler to teenager).

And this one I just love to bits:

'Well, of course I didn't like it. Pip was standing a few feet away from me as I was reading it. (Pip and I are working at Fawley Refinery for the next three weeks). I told her what you'd just told me, then burst out laughing. Which I think she thought terribly callous of me. But it was your description of the endangered species on the ceiling and your brush with the healthcare system that did it.

'And if you happen to like Abba music (it divides the population into two of course) buy the DVD of *Mamma Mia* which even this man can see is the ultimate feelgood movie of all time. At least three of my friends watch it when they feel a bit down. It's so good to see a movie (hugely successful at that) that centres around three middle-aged women. If it appeals, have it on really loud (a 5.1 sound system is ideal) and belt out 'Waterloo' so they can hear it in Brodie.

'I'll have to think again if you hate Abba.' David Taylor (Aurora Perceptions and other stuff – we meet for coffee often – might have to be at my house next time.)

I got the *Mama Mia* DVD for Christmas from my Mum; I now have the soundtrack from Jim. It saves watching the DVD and working at the same time and when driving the car it's safer, doesn't have 'Waterloo' though.

Chocolate porridge time, I think . . .

NLP stuff: Words

Remember I mentioned earlier, NLP is a communication model about human behaviours, and by using it successfully we can 'run our own brain' (and that means our emotions or feelings as they are often called), and we can create more resourcefulness and therefore find it easier to work on finding and putting into practice our highest potentials and possibilities.

Well, I also mentioned in that last diary excerpt: 'By the way words like 'rough', 'tough', 'problem', 'difficult', 'illness' etc. are banned'. Why? Well, to me they are all exhausting, like the 'battle' with cancer, the 'fight', the 'struggle', has 'overcome cancer'. Now, I've decided there will no battling here, and no struggling, and no problems, or I'll be tired out.

Think about it, when 'life is hard' and 'it's an uphill struggle' and the 'weight of the world is on my shoulders' and there are only 'problems' and it's 'tough', when it's a 'bad' day, it all 'looks black' – what happens?

Now think about 'good times, things 'being easier', 'there's a way round it all', 'it's a piece of cake' (perhaps not because I am on a diet), 'I want to move forwards'/'I want to avoid this at all costs' – what's that like?

And if you are saying 'well it's alright for you' – believe me it was not alright for me, but – and it's a huge whacking great BUT – I have two grandsons and I want to spend more time with them, and I have a plan and by now I know have a Compelling Purpose (more on that later). You may not think you have a future and the 'medical model' at times puts a huge damper on that, but you do have a future, you can create a future, a future that's compelling.

So I changed my language and I slapped my own fingers (figuratively, of course) and I became even more positive (annoyingly positive, someone told me, for my state of health) and sadly for some people I cut them out of my life, I ignored what they said (as it wasn't useful for me and some of it was factually incorrect) and I didn't go back for a second helping of dispiriting language (one of them follows in the next diary excerpt). Some people I told, especially every single person or who knows something about NLP who emailed me or said something to me in that vein, I reminded them 'that's your model, that's the way you see it, you talk about it, you feel about it and THIS IS ME and I want to be well and cancer free'. So I asked: 'why does it have to be difficult?', 'why is it hard?'. It was not easy, and it was a bumpy journey and I noticed that, and I said to myself, 'I want things to be easier for me,' 'I want a result that is good for me,' 'I want to avoid pain (and radiotherapy, you're not grilling me)', 'I want to live forever, light up the sky with my name!'

NLP stuff: Words and wheelbarrows

NLP talks about how we shape our world (you know we don't live in reality? That we form our own idea of reality?). In doing this we delete, distort and generalise.

Alfred Korzybski, the founder of general semantics, found that language functions in the human nervous system as a map or blueprint of reality. Language is purely a symbolic system and therefore it's never reality. To deal with the world we select information, interpret it in our way and use this information as our map to negotiate our way through life – to do this we use Distort, Delete and Generalise in the language that we use.

Richard Bandler and John Grinder (the co-developers of NLP) developed the Meta Model chiefly from the Gestalt therapy of Fritz Perls and the work of the internationally famous family therapist Virginia Satir and used this in their book *The Structure of Magic I*. They developed fourteen linguistic distinctions which are used to indicate how language shows ill-formedness (not saying what we really mean, using short-cut language) from the way in which Perls and Satir 'challenged' the Deletions, Distortions, and Generalisations, to recover what we really mean when we speak or write something. After all, the words are the tip of the iceberg in a conversation.

Now I'm not writing about all fourteen linguistic distinctions, just about one of the Deletions which are known in NLP as 'Nominalisations'.

People nominalise things in order to make understanding/meaning out of them, or to refer to them in simpler terms. We produce nouns describing a state of being which exists in name only, so they are not a tangible item (i.e. Fulfilment, Peace, Oneness, Existence, Divinity), they can be a verb or another process word that has been formed into a noun (i.e. Decision, Realisation, Thought). It's easier to deal with when we turn it back into the process.

An example: a word like 'Relationship'

First, it can have so many meanings – it can be a relationship with a significant other, with a friend, with a child, with a customer, with a client, with a work colleague, with a boss etc. And whatever of those it is, it can have completely different meanings to those people involved in the relationship (or not).

So when someone says 'my relationship is not right', we really need to start asking that person questions, not assuming we know what they are talking about. After all, we only know about the kind of relationships we are in, or the ones we have known, or seen from our perspective. If we assume and give our advice, the worst-case scenario is that we can lose a friend or be blamed for giving advice that was well meaning, but they may not have wanted that advice.

To find out more about what a word means for the other person, we need to turn that nominalisation into a process and find out what's not right for the person who made the statement 'my relationship is not right'. So we ask (carefully, with great respect and sincerity and in a kind of the 'pass the salt' tone) something like 'how would you like to be related to?' It might seem weird, but this will give you more to work with. It might bring up another nominalisation or other deletions, distortions and generalisations, but I only wanted to give you this as a taster. You will then find you have more idea of what the person means (and you could have been barking up the wrong tree) and their relationship, and what also eventually happens is that the person who was having the problem has more idea of what it is they want in life.

However, we need some clues to which words are nominalisations. There's the wheelbarrow mentioned in the title. There's a kind of rule of thumb that anything you couldn't put in a wheelbarrow (and sometimes it will be a very large wheelbarrow, for example, for a 'crowd', a 'building' etc.) is a nominalisation, so things like 'fear', 'love', 'hate' etc. and also words ending in the following:

-ance (e.g. compliance)

-iency (e.g. efficiency)

-ful (e.g. painful)

-ship (e.g. friendship)

-able (e.g. reliable)

-ness (e.g. happiness)

-itude (e.g. gratitude)

-ment (e.g. fulfilment)

-ence (e.g. difference)

-ion (e.g. depression)

Now you can apply the kind of questioning I mentioned earlier; sometimes it's not so obvious what the process word/doing word/verb is, sometimes we just need to think a little about how we will ask a question to get to the root or heart of the matter, so that we understand more about what the other person is annoyed or upset or aggrieved about. So the following are all examples you could use (there are others):

Compliance: How's that not complied with? or How would you like that to be complied with?

Efficiency: How do we need to be more efficient?

Painful: Tell me more about the pain.

Friendship: How would you expect a friend to be? or Tell me more about being friends.

Reliable: What would someone you can rely on be like?

Happiness: How would you like to be happy?

Gratitude: How would you like them to be grateful?

Fulfilment: How would you like them to be fulfilled?

Difference: How do they differ?

Depression: How does that depress you?

This kind of thing is really useful. What is also useful and helps you avoid the pain of misunderstanding and misinterpreting and losing friendships, preventing the onset of World War III at home, getting to the core of a problem at work, is thinking in this way:

Notice how you form your own reality, pay attention to what you are saying to yourself – this will make you more effective and successful. Also think about what you say to others: if you are not clear, if you use lots of nominalisations (and some cultures and organisations do, all the time) how will others understand you?

Always be in rapport (so point your body towards the person, match or mirror their posture, use their words), soften your voice and phrase questions in a more acceptable way.

'I wonder exactly what you mean by that . . .'

'That's interesting, can I ask you . . .'

Think carefully about what you say and listen carefully to what others say and train your intuition to recognise patterns, know when there's information missing, when it's useful to clarify meaning or open choices. Where the conversation is based on a relationship (of whatever kind), be careful, very, very careful with the Meta Model – if not used with care it becomes a task-based process. For example if someone says 'I liked that', asking 'How specifically did you like it and what exactly did you like?' may not be appropriate in certain circumstances, and I can think of a few ☺

4th February 2009: Oh doctors

It's Wednesday 4th February today, the day before my little brother's birthday (I've told him in his birthday card that I've got cancer). The M-day[3] is 26th February, I found out on Monday this week.

Monday got to be exhausting, you know, one of 'those days', me cancelling things and explaining to other people, not least one of our GPs. I'm changing my GP. Unfortunately we have two surgeries here locally and both have the same admin (they have done various things with my appointments and other stuff recently). The icing on the cake in January was from someone in the admin staff, and then another doctor, telling me they had prescribed me some antibiotics (and I'm still unclear why, and the way it was done was appalling) and that I must not drink alcohol (well, I replied 'that's not a problem, I don't drink alcohol': 'are you sure' they both asked (you know the phrase 'red rag to a bull'?). Of course I'm sure I don't drink – some of my family call me boring.

Anyway, I have to be reassigned as I'm out of the area for the other surgeries. I tried Nairn but the person who answered the phone was 'snippy'. I've opted for an Elgin practice cos both the

---

[3] Mastectomy Day

person who answered the phone (we don't get people in Forres) and the practice manager were really nice!!

My GP in Forres on Monday left a message on our answer phone: she was phoning 'about the arrangements for Rosie'. (I wondered, had I died? Was I in a parallel universe?)

To cut a long story short, I actually got to speak to her. What came across was that she was apologising on behalf of the practice and worried I might be complaining or something and was at great pains to point out that the mammogram had detected the cancer early and that I had to be grateful for that, but she also waffled on about I was ill, I must realise I was very ill! And it would be an idea to stop working now. (Has she met me when I'm bored?)

Anyway, her talk which was all about her and how she would feel (flipping hypochondriacs, some of these doctors) and not about me (definite need for NLP skills in the NHS: State Maintenance and Second Positioning (see next chapter), respect of other person, Model of the World) and I was so cool, calm and collected and she had a problem with me being positive. I HATE THIS.

I AM NOT ILL – I HAVE A LUMP, AND I AM A BIT TIRED – YES AND I COULD GET VERY GRUMPY – I AM DOING LYING DOWN (MORE OFTEN THAN FOR A LONG TIME) AND I HAVEN'T GONE

TO INVERNESS TODAY AS JOANNA CAN MANAGE WITHOUT ME.

LIFE WILL GO ON AND I WILL BE PRESENTING ON 19TH MARCH IN ABERDEEN ALONGSIDE THE HEAD OF MICROSOFT SECURITY IN THE UK – COS THAT'S WHAT I CALL A COMPELLING PURPOSE!

And wickedly, I'm looking forward to testing the state maintenance of twelve people at the weekend in Aberdeen!

It's very tiring when I get comments like 'Sorry you are going through a tough time'. And then people proceed to tell me about their experiences of something, this is not helpful, I don't want to know how I feel (with my hands is our usual family answer) and I want to stay away from other people putting me in a place I'm avoiding (you know that scenario, someone tells you you look ill etc. and up until then you had been fine?). I only want experiences that tell me you can get rid of this stuff by alternative measures – haven't found anyone – yet!

These came this morning via Facebook, I've known April and her daughters Berni and Tiggy for 30 years and in spite of a gap of 15 years and just meeting up last year on Facebook again – this is what they have to say:

'Hi Rosie. Don't get on computer much but just had 10 mins to spare and got your news. That's shit news but I know how strong you are and that you won't stand for any of it. My thoughts and prayers are with you. **I know you'll be fine.** love April' (Hermion, Wales)

'Hi Rosie, I'm really sorry to hear that, what a nightmare! I'm guessing you're not gonna let it get u down tho, **the Rosie I remember is way too strong for that!** Keep in touch. My love and thoughts are with you. Berni xxx' (New Zealand)

'Oh, Rosie. All my thoughts and love are sent with this message. I do hear they can do amazing things for **'Mr. C'** nowadays, please keep us posted. All our love Tiggy, Geoff and baby Tomas xxx' (Hertfordshire)

(The bold bits are what give me strength – hey ho, Mr C.)

This is also a useful reaction for me:

'Hi Rosie

'Back online and so sorry to hear about your **unexpected challenge** Rosie. Don't worry at all about the 2nd/3rd March, and please focus all your energies on recovering well!

'If once you're back in action, you'd still like to speak to the group in Oban, the next dates are 24–25th March (Tuesday–Wednesday) and you would be welcomed.

'Look after yourself, all best wishes, and get in touch in due course if it suits.

'And by the way we are still having sex (why not)! And I'm already considering what alternative positions there are for after the op!'

NLP stuff: State Maintenance and Second Positioning

The medical world needs NLP skills – State Maintenance and Second Positioning, respect of other person, Model of the World. Well guys, it's true.

State maintenance means maintaining a good and useful state for me and the other person I am interacting with. And that means:

I need to get a good and resourceful state, see NLP stuff on good and useful state, when I am working with somebody or just being with somebody. Sometimes, part of that is about breathing. Another part is about checking 'am I ok?' and 'if I'm not I need to get into a good and resourceful state'. The Circle of Excellence is a good way, see below.

I need to put my Model of the World (what I know and believe to be true, what I have experienced in my life) on one side.

I need to have rapport, and I need to listen to that person.

I need to be respectful of that person and what they know and believe to be true.

I need to be genuine about it as well.

And then and only then I need to use my experience and knowledge and skills and capabilities to get that person to where it is most useful for that person to be and to get the best result for that person.

Let me explain Second Positioning.

Well, when I'm being me I'm in First Position, that's when I put me first, and my job and my schedule and sometimes that includes the department I work in as I become a part of that and it consumes me. When I'm in Second Position, I'm there for the other person, I'm watching listening and guiding them, I'm putting my own stuff on one side. If I start deciding I know what's best (based on whatever I know and believe to be true), I'm disregarding the other person and I'm being in First Position. It's good idea to be in Second Position when you want to help usefully. We know from our experience of everyday life, that not everyone shares our point of view; so in order to understand a situation fully it's useful to take on different perspectives, just as if you were viewing an object from different angles to get an idea of its width, height and length. So for example, being in Second Position is about understanding things from the other person's point of view 'being in their shoes as them' and using some good listening skills). It's not useful to be in Second Position all the time as you will forget to look after yourself, so it takes some working on and it's great when you get there – believe me.There's also a Third or Meta Position – that's when you hop out of your head and look at the situation as if you were a fly on the wall or in a helicopter – or for me – I'm a Terry Pratchett fan – you're Granny Weatherwax!). I will mention both Third Position and Terry Pratchett again later.

The Circle of Excellence technique

1. Stand up and think back to a time when you were very confident, you achieved something really good. Relive that moment, seeing what you see, hearing what you hear and feeling what you feel.

Briefly think about something else,

like what did you have for breakfast (or should you have had)?

2. Relive that moment, see what you see, with any colours, any pictures, any scenery, any people and anything that was around, only you can know what this was, hear what you hear, any sounds that are particularly important to this time, anything you said to yourself or someone else said to you, as appropriate for this 'wow' experience and then finally, feel what you feel at that time, where are the feelings, in your body, all around you.

Briefly think about something else,

like what did you have for lunch (or should you have had)?

3. Go back and experience all of that again and then turn it all up, the sights, the sounds, the feelings, as if you have a remote control or a dial or a slide bar on a computer screen – turn it all up as far as is still comfortable.

Briefly think about something else, like your phone number backwards.

4. As you feel the confidence building up inside you, imagine a circle on the floor just in front of you and colour this in with whatever colour you like.

Does it need to have a sound as well that indicates how powerful it is (only you can hear the sound)? Step into that circle taking all the sights, sounds and feelings with you.

When that feeling of confidence is at its fullest, step out of that circle, leaving those extra confident feelings that you want to build up for the future inside the circle.

Briefly think about something else, like your phone number backwards.

5. Now think of a time in your future when you want to have that same feeling of confidence. See and hear what will be there just before you want to feel confident. This could be the door of a meeting room, answering the phone etc.

6. As soon as these cues are clear in your mind, step back into the circle and feel those confident feelings. Imagine that situation unfolding around you in the future with these confident feelings fully available to you.

Now step out of the circle again, leaving the extra confident feelings in the circle. Whilst outside, take a moment to think of that event in the future. Those confident feelings will come to you automatically. You've already reprogrammed yourself for that future event. You're feeling better about it and it hasn't even happened. When it does, you will naturally respond more confidently.

If you find that difficult, here are some tips:

If the difficulty is in finding a really wow moment, can you think of someone you know and admire who is really confident? They could be a real person, or TV, or film character (if you have any children you might use this circle for confidence and use Harry Potter, Tracy Beaker or whoever else is their positive idol) and create what that character will be seeing, hearing and feeling in the same way.

If stepping into the circle is an issue, then once you've got that supreme state, see a colour in front of you and touch the seam on your trousers or skirt just as you get to the peak time and know that you can do that any time you want to, to get this state of confidence back again. Or other things you can do are imagine you are stepping through a doorway or arch, switching spotlights on.

It works, you have to practise though and you can do this in the privacy of your own home, and practise often, only 'perfect practice makes perfect' you know.

I've done this now for years and I have a 'one size fits all' circle that I use for many occasions, usually when meeting people in business situations or presenting and sometimes when meeting people in social situations especially if I would rather be somewhere else. But you can have a circle for each different occasion, if you want, you can chain circles together.

1st February 2009: To detox or not to detox

One of my friends asked me about detoxing and sent me a link to an article on the web which advocates detoxing. This was my reply to him:

'Now the whole detox thing seems so wrong to me, why deplete your body at a time when it's not doing so well any way?

'In 2004 I went on a detox programme from a naturopath – it nearly finished me off and made me really ill, when I was possibly fairly well – so I view this stuff with great scepticism. Another thing is that a homeopath told me some complete tosh recently in respect of progesterone and oestrogen when she got it the wrong way round and then bought supposed information to back up what she had said up (as in a colleague of hers and someone at the college agreed with her, so that I am even more wary of too many alternatives – perhaps the 'gut feeling' is appropriate here).'

However, I sent my friend a Word file of Brodie's *The Cancer Personality* (some of it is quoted in the next chapter), I downloaded this last summer in respect of something else, it's very interesting, particularly the highlighted pieces.

'Reading this and taking it onboard (and I have subsequently checked this out with several people who give it credence), then I know where the cancer came from, it makes sense, you can remember the event [I wrote to him].

'It's at early stage this cancer of mine – can I afford to mess with it as in hoping that a natural cure will work and then perhaps make it worse? I've yet to meet someone who has come through cancer using alternative methods, no one talks about it if they have. I do know that I have been taking medication which may have aggravated it [it turns out the oestrogen I was taking would have fed the tumour and encouraged it to grow but not started its growth], and I also know that the stress I went through in respect of all my daughters last year won't have helped – I am letting lots of things go – I've also stopped taking the stuff my homeopath sent me (and I feel much better) and am cooking a castor oil poultice in the oven.

'I got a very good book (*Breast Cancer? Breast Health!*) in Findhorn yesterday in which the author gives you all the pros and cons and leaves you to make up your own mind – she has thoroughly researched breasts and cancer and women and she is a woman – she respects that some people will want and have surgery and some not and she gives a more sensible idea of what I see as a healthy and useful diet that coupled with some understanding will work I believe.

'I also, through her, know now of some possible options but I need to know more about the diagnosis to explore these.

'One of the best pieces of advice I was given came from a woman I met at a Day Care Centre in Inverness. She by then had secondary cancer. 'Don't read too much' she said, 'you will get conflicting advice'. She was right, not only that but some of the stuff then becomes psychosomatic (you start to think you have that or should have that, you start to worry).' (More on that later.)

The cancer personality

Written sometime between 4th and 12th February 2009, this one did not go out to the diary recipients!

My Mum phoned me last Friday, my Mum rarely phones, she uses email [will be 80 this year] – oh Mum I wish you'd phoned me in 2005!

I believe that my cancer is attributable to this.

Now important is there is no blame, it's a set of circumstances, but maybe, just maybe if some people had supported me better, or I had coped better, in this particular shit things might have been different . . .

Read here from *The Cancer Personality* (www.alternative-cancer-care.com), W Douglas Brodie, MD:

'In dealing with many thousands of cancer patients over the past 28 years, it has been my observation that there are certain personality traits which are rather consistently present in the cancer-susceptible individual. These characteristics are as follows:

'1. Being highly conscientious, dutiful, responsible, caring, hardworking, and usually of above average intelligence.

'2. Exhibiting a strong tendency toward carrying other people's burdens and toward taking on extra obligations, often "worrying for others."

'3. Having a deep-seated need to make others happy, tending to be "people pleasers." Having a great need for approval.

'These people have a tremendous need for approval and acceptance, developing a very high sensitivity to the needs of others while suppressing their own emotional needs.

'These good folks become the "caretakers" of the world, showing great compassion and caring for others, and going out of their way to look after the needs of others. They are very reluctant to accept help from others, fearing that it may jeopardize their role as caretakers or that they might appear to have too much self-concern. Throughout their childhood they have typically been taught "not to be selfish," and they take this to heart as a major lifetime objective. All of this benevolence is highly commendable, of course, in our culture, but must be somehow modified in the case of the cancer patient. A distinction needs to be made here between the "care-giving" and the "care-taking" personality. There is nothing wrong with care-giving, of course, but the problem arises when the susceptible individual derives his/her entire worth, value and identity from his/her role as "caretaker."

'Most cancer patients have experienced a highly stressful event, usually about 2 years prior to the onset of detectable disease. This traumatic event is often beyond the patient's control, such as the loss of a loved one, loss of a business, job, home, or some other major disaster. The typical cancer victim has lost the ability to cope with these extreme events, because his/her coping mechanism lies in his/her ability to control the environment. When this control is lost, the patient has no other way to cope.

'Major stress, as we have seen, causes suppression of the immune system, and does so more overwhelmingly in the cancer-susceptible individual than in others. Thus personal tragedies and excessive levels of stress appear to combine with the underlying personality described above to bring on the immune deficiency which allows cancer to thrive.

'Those susceptible to cancer, are highly vulnerable to life's stresses and trauma, and feel unable to cope when life throws a curve-ball their way. These people are perfectionists and live in fear of conflict, stress, trauma and loss and are deeply frightened of negative events "happening" to them. And when faced with a highly stressful or traumatic event they have not anticipated, which inevitably happens during their life, react adversely and are unable to cope.

'They experience Inescapable Shock and remain deeply affected by the experience. They have difficulty in expressing their inner grief, their inner pain, their inner anger or resentment, and genuinely feel there is no way out of the pain they are feeling inside. And because their mind cannot fathom what has happened, and remains in a state of disbelief or denial, these inner painful feelings are continually perpetuated, shooting up stress levels, lowering melatonin and adrenaline levels, causing a slow breakdown of the emotional reflex centre in the brain, and creating the beginning of cancer progression in the body.

'When faced with a major trauma, the cancer personality feels trapped and unable to escape from the memory of the traumatic experience and the painful feelings of the experience. Stress hormone cortisol levels skyrocket and remain at high levels, directly suppressing the immune system, whose job it is to destroy cancer cells that exist in every human being. High stress levels generally means a person cannot sleep well, and cannot produce enough Melatonin during deep sleep. Melatonin is responsible for inhibiting cancer cell growth. This means cancer cells are now free to multiply. Adrenaline levels also skyrocket initially, but are then drained and depleted over time. This is especially bad news for the cancer personality.

'Adrenaline is responsible for transporting sugar away from cells. And when there is no adrenaline left, sugar builds up in cells of the body. Viral-bacterial-yeast-like-fungus then inhabit normal cells to feed on this excess sugar, breaking the cell's (oxygen) krebs cycle. This means normal body cells cannot breathe properly because of low oxygen and mutate during the dividing process into cancer cells. Cancer cells thrive in a low

50

oxygen state, as demonstrated by Nobel Prize winner Otto Warburg. Cancer cells also thrive on fermented sugar for cell division, and this is provided by the viral-bacterial-yeast-like-fungus that ferment and feed on sugar in the perfect symbiotic relationship.

'Put simply, too much internal stress causes a depletion of adrenaline, leads to too much sugar in the body's cells, resulting in the perfect environment for cancer cells to thrive in the body.'

I'm not quite sure when 'the onset was' but one November day in 2005 I got on a train from London Kings Cross to Inverness and I phoned my son to say I was on my way home, and meet you at the station. Then the battery on the phone went dead, and there were no sockets to charge the phone on that train. When I arrived in Inverness, eventually I discovered a taxi driver was waiting for me with an envelope with the house key and a note – and my son was gone!

Words like 'devastated' and 'angry' were not enough – he did some silly things, but the not knowing was the worst. My life this time fell apart. It was worse than being beaten up by Klaus (my son's father), it was worse than Michael (my second husband) dying. Where the hell was Jacob?

The oddest support came from my odd friend Les Cameron, who supported me in the way he knew how.

The sterling support came from my daughter Kristin on the phone almost every evening. I spent Christmas Day, and Boxing Day,

and the days in between,

and Hogmanay,

and New Year's Day,

and the days after that

on my own,

hoping, hoping that my son would phone

or someone would phone

and tell me where he was.

What still fascinates me is that neither my parents nor my brother phoned me over that time, I asked my mother why she didn't phone, she said 'she didn't know what to say'. Hello? They didn't even phone on Christmas Day or New Year's Day.

I did a lot of wall climbing at that time, well it certainly felt like it!

When my son reappeared, I happened to be in London going to a course. He didn't know what to say to me and I just wanted to know why. Subsequently, he spent time with parents, and my brother, and none of them spoke to me.

Hey guys do you know how much that hurt? And I still don't know why.

Now, it doesn't matter: I saw J last September in Nuremberg with his girlfriend and things are good for him.

However, Dr Brodie goes on to mention one of the most recent studies on psychosomatic cancer therapy from the German medical doctor and cancer surgeon Ryke-Geerd Hamer. Over the past ten years, he has examined 20,000 cancer patients with all types of cancer and, according to Dr Hamer, the real cause of cancer and other diseases is an unexpected traumatic shock for which we are emotionally unprepared. He lists some of the relationships between conflict emotions and target organs.

And what does it say relating to me?

Breast (Left)	Conflict Concerning Child, Home, or Mother

It's really odd I read all this last year in respect of something else.

LIFE GOES ON.

I started concentrating on my Compelling Purpose – this was to be presenting 'Creating a Compelling Purpose' to the Girl Geek Dinner in Aberdeen on 19th March. When I agreed to do this (actually mid-January, but the date was confirmed on 26th January) I had no idea the proceeds were to go to Breast Cancer Care! It's my Compelling Purpose to be there, I'll be a little breastless on the night (that's Jim's phrase) ☺ and I'm going there to inspire me, never mind anyone else ;

I've trained for 2 days on my Aberdeen Practitioner course. Seven out of twelve turned up, some managed to say why they were not there, and some did not. I acknowledge there was some snow around! The (magnificent) seven all maintained a good and useful state when I explained why Rebecca (ah, Rebecca what would I do without you?) would be there instead of me (and I told them they must be good to her on the feedback forms) in March. It actually evoked lots of discussion and work around healing, using Milton Language[4] and please hope that Ania doesn't undergo some horrible disfiguring operation on her saliva gland, but uses NLP to diminish the size of the lumps in her neck and throat! Please hope that Susan gets her friend who has had a mastectomy to speak to her! [Susan did contact her friend! Ania had the op.]

My Pilates instructor, Sara, called me 'Treasure' when I phoned her last night to change my class from morning to afternoon so that I get home to Forres safely. We've had a lot of snow in Aberdeen and I want other people to have driven on the road before I leave here.

So I'll go and rest now.

---

[4] I.e., the language of trance of Milton Erikson.

NLP stuff: Creating a compelling purpose

Think about what you want and make an image of it, out in front of you, either as a picture or something panoramic (no frame). Add colour to that image and add absolutely anything into that image that you want to happen.

So for me it was presenting to 70 people, 3 weeks to the day after my op. I already knew the room I would be presenting in, so imagined it full of 70 people, mainly women in this case, lots of different colours there and I saw a man in a dark suit, the other presenter and I saw me. Me with my hair newly coloured and done by the hairdresser, me in a new red jacket and brown trousers.

I heard someone introducing me, I heard myself speaking and I heard applause at the end of it.

And I felt how I would feel at the end of my 15 minute presentation, a good warm feeling in my stomach that I had stood up there.

So I saw all of this happening, and I heard it in surround sound, and I felt it in every cell of my body. And it happened like that. I practised this happening before I went into hospital and I built the image up with the things I could see and the sounds I could hear and the feelings I could feel and I pulled this image towards me and I stepped into all of this and I checked out what it would be like.

Now if you think this is difficult and that you can't do it, that you can't see things, start from the sense that is easiest for you, feel how it will feel for you or hear what you will hear, what you are saying or what others are saying, and then add the parts from the seeing or the feeling. Practise and practise adding bits in, until you can get this whole sensory experience in your mind. It's important that you add elements from all the senses. I once had a course participant who set this kind of Compelling Purpose up and I listened in, whilst she and someone else worked together and I noticed something was missing, so asked the person working with her, 'What's missing?'. He thought a little and said 'she wants to set up a client-based business, which requires clients to come into her office and there are no people in what she is seeing, everything else is there.' Yes and she said she 'couldn't put the people in there, as she didn't know who they were'. This was in May, and do you know what? By December she had given up her business!

Another thing, is your language holding you back?

What happens when you change your language sometimes?

For example, try changing a phrase like:

From 'I can't do this'   *to* 'I won't do this'

From 'I know they'll be'   *to* 'I imagine they'll be . . .'

From 'I have to be here'   *to* 'I choose to be here'

From 'I must do this now'   *to* 'I want to do this now'

Eventually you'll give yourself more options and eventually you will find things easier to do, or things easier to say no to.

12nd February 2009: My state maintenance slipped

If I still believed in God at this precise moment in time this morning, I would say . . . there is one. I just logged into my bank account to find out if my tax refund was there – and it is – and it will cover all my expenses for the next couple of months – thanks really to Mark wot does my books – a weight off my mind – yippee. (I took a lot of time off last year – it's called work–life balance).

Well, my state maintenance went yesterday. As you already know, a prerequisite to becoming an NLP Practitioner (and I'm the trainer) is maintaining a good and useful state for you and the other person (or persons). Well my state maintenance went big time yesterday – now I notice that's not useful, cos I get upset and I ache. Partially it went due to the fact that until just now (cos I finished my next set of accounts paperwork about 10 mins ago) there was lots of clutter, then there was something I read that I didn't particularly like. Then I read some tripe from someone very dear to me, I had no idea why they were reacting badly – now I realise they are having a problem cos of my cancer, 'scuse me!

Now this is important if you are around someone with cancer: your problems in respect of that person's cancer are so totally unuseful and so totally unimportant to the person who has cancer. We need your support (after all in 2 weeks my underwired bras will be no good on the left, will they?) so, all the support we can get. Now flaming well ask the cancer patient, whoever we are 'What can I do to help you?' How you would handle it and how you feel is sooooo unimportant and frankly shite, cos I have cancer, not you.

Mind you, if your cancer person is me, other people's problems and my work keeps my mind off all the rubbish that whirls around in my life – I've no idea how others get on with their lives, but bet your bottom dollar I will have an NLP model, a book and other stuff on how to do this – there's a silver lining to every cloud.

I had lost it big time yesterday with Scottish Electricity and their bullying way of getting new business, oh wait 'til I get hold of them and a few other people on the way. Mind you the pleasure in getting the Yellow Pages guy off the phone (they are trained to ignore the word 'no'): I got rid of him by saying 'I am having my left breast cut off in 2 weeks, do you really think I want to talk about advertising?' That was immensely satisfying and maybe he learned something – well I live in hope!

Anyway, around 3 p.m. Rebecca (yes it's her again) phoned to ask me where I was (I was supposed to be in Inverness). This reminded me to get my act together and I went off to Inverness. On walking out of the car park in Inverness, I realised I'd left the key to the Practice Group Venue at home (lawks). However I had, on putting the car parking ticket in the back pocket of my handbag which I never use, discovered my mobile phone (the new one) that I thought I'd lost the day before – ah. According to my middle daughter-in-law (there's no shorter way to describe the relationship) and in her father's words 'You get to be like the folk you bide with!' At this point, please know I have done this before with the phone, and once with my purse and all my various money cards (they were under a pile of the books on the desk for 3 days!) – misplacing things has nothing to do with my present state of dis-ease – it's called trance, we are all in a trance at some time. Have you ever asked yourself 'who ate the other half of my biscuit?' and you're the only one around!

Rebecca and I had a sumptuous and healthy tea in the Mustard Seed in Inverness – mmm. Then we went to off to check my car hadn't been locked in the car park and go to the venue to make an action plan – ah when we got there, the blessed Tara goddess of compassion, and several hundred guardian angels had kept the cleaner there (drives an Audi TT and lives in a very posh new house – where there's dirt, there's money, noted for later if I change my job) and she loaned me her key. So have the phone and have the venue – five lovely ladies turned up (why, guys, can't you get off your bums and learn something about doing things differently?) And we had a great time visualising and listening out for and feeling about compelling outcomes ☺ Rebecca and I found where the cleaner lived and dropped the key off and I got home on a roll.

Have ordered the breast casting kit!

Oh yes, outside it's snowing again, lovely perhaps I'll get the camera out later and I hope choir is still on tonight. I have long johns (bought them in Germany to watch to the Dons – Aberdeen football team – when playing in Aberdeen at the baltic Pittodrie Stadium).

Off to do my Pilates now ☺

By the way, in 1993 a group of scientists led by John Hagelin conducted an experiment in which several thousand people in Washington DC would meditate together twice a day for almost 2 months. This was correlated with a highly significant reduction in crime in DC.

You don't have to meditate but send me Good Vibrations (anybody have that by the Beach Boys?) and to anyone else – when we radiate out good vibrations we will get them back.

Perception is projection ☺ Have a wonderful day.

NLP stuff: Dealing with an incident from the past

What did I do about the incident about my son, in respect of this cancer I had?

Well, I did two things:

1. I went into First Position (acted just as me, thinking about me) – I had the cancer.

2. I looked at his emails and I recognised, whilst in Second Position, there were things about what he had said that were unclear, he'd left bits out (deletion), he'd generalised and distorted. Yes, he was upset.

And I realised I can be Mummy (but er, he's 28) and help him sort himself out, or I can make the decision to say 'sorry I don't want to know, and I do want to live and get well'.

Now, for a long time I had had this 'wanting to know why he had done this disappearing in 2005?', 'why my Mum and brother wouldn't tell me anything (if they actually knew anything)', 'why, why, why'. Also since then, sleeping all night was a very rare occurrence for me (at this point I hadn't linked these two things).

So I thought to myself, I need to deal with this, so I used an NLP technique, Change Personal History.[5] This is what is called a change process that is good for recurring problem behaviours or emotions. It uses a 'timeline' and so helps you to go back through time to access a problem in the past that is causing problems in the present.

I made sure I was in a good and resourceful state. (I was laid in bed at the time, early in the morning on my right side – not particularly relevant but it was like that)

I thought (briefly) about 'wanting to know why he had done this?', 'why my Mum and brother wouldn't tell me anything (if they actually knew anything)', 'why, why, why'. And that this was what I wanted to change. I experienced it and noticed where I sensed it in my body.

I know I represent my future out to the front of me, slightly to the right and my past is out to my left side. I made sure I was mentally in the present (so thinking about the here and now). I recreated this sensation I had been having and I pressed on my right shoulder with my left hand (NLP calls this 'anchoring' in the present). And I 'walked back in my mind' towards the past, focussing my attention on what had happened for me and I noticed any memories or associations that came up for me. I was doing this 'seeing what I was seeing', 'hearing what I was hearing' and 'feeling what I was feeling', as if it was happening now.

I was experiencing myself becoming younger and younger and noticed (in my mind's eye) what I was experiencing. Going back to my earliest memory of that sensation.

---

[5] Change Personal History was developed by Bandler and Grinder. The term comes from computing and Change History is the term used for the record of corrections made to the program or user's manual. Thanks to Robert Dilts for this material.

When I came to that memory in 2005, I stepped off the timeline (in my mind's eye and you can do this physically) and looked at the timeline from the present day as an observer.

I told myself I had done the best I could at that time in that situation and with the resources and knowledge I had available to me at the time. I know now that I am even more mature and have additional resources and knowledge available to me now. (We all have resources, things that we can do, strengths that are useful for ourselves and others).

For me, I thought about my strengths and how I enable other people to change and improve and to bring about change and improvement. I thought about my achievements in life before that, and after that, and I made all of that into a soft ball-like shape of energy which I took back to me at that time. I stepped back on the timeline with this soft ball-like shape of energy and walked slowly back to the present and 'Changed History', changing and updating the events, with this soft ball-like shape of energy as a new resource (everything combined together what power and strength) to the present and I noticed along the way how my memories and perceptions of events had changed.

I no longer 'need to know'. I've been back and forgiven myself for all the things I didn't' understand and possible failings I may have had and I've 'blessed' J and let him go to get on with his own life. (And since the op, I can now sleep all night!)

Fantastic! Trainer, get your own act together ☺

16th February 2009: Getting plastered

I'm a little uncertain why my mind is racing at 4-ish in the morning. Maybe I'm a little hot due to my hormones, maybe it's because I needed to get up to read over a dozen reasons a course participant is giving me for something that I don't understand (she missed a weekend), so is she now setting herself up to fail her assessment or duck out of the whole course? I never cease to be amazed at how people can come up with detailed reasons and be completely unspecific as to what they want from you! It's often best to let that go, as eventually they sort themselves out. [September 2010: I can say about the lady in question, she had a lot on her mind and has since changed her life and put all her Compelling Purposes into action and has more to come ☺]

Anyway, it's 10 days and counting down to 'M-day'. I actually read the leaflet on what to expect in hospital and after surgery, just before sitting down at my desk. Oh well, the sooner I get in and out the better.

I went to choir on Thursday, it was good and I went to a singing session on Saturday and afterwards out 'for coffee' with some of the guys and gals from choir, that was good and made a change from working all weekend. Then bumped into a couple of neighbours and a mad foreign guy locally, who regaled me with this woes, which is why I like to keep away from him and his tales of 'no one listens to me'. I wonder why? ☺

Then I got back home just before a friend came round for a short while, and she left when some fella phoned her. Oh ladies, girls, women, you don't just rush off when they call. In my experience, that behaviour is symptomatic of a relationship either that's an 'affair' or there is something there about the relationship that the woman refuses to admit is 'wrong'. Trust me.

Yesterday I got plastered.

My friend Rebecca came round on Sunday [I was a bowls widow – Jim was playing bowls, at the weekend, 'again' as Leon would say] and together (I work better when someone reads me the instructions, I remembered), using the casting kit,[6] Rebecca and I made a rubber mould over my left boob. Then we covered the rubber mould in plaster bandages and after it had dried out and become hard, I took the 'casting mould' as it now was, off the boob and we propped it up on some telephone directories and we made up three lots of plaster mix, each time a little thicker and poured that in the mould. It involved lots of hilarity, and towels and plastic on the floor (those were in the copious instructions). And it's one of

---

[6] www.bodycast-studio.co.uk for plaster casting kit with all instructions.

those occasions when you seriously hope no one will phone or come round (in case you have to explain!). Fascinating.

I now have a plaster cast boob resplendent on my kitchen table. It took ages; we had lunch and tea together. It was great to have Rebecca there, as always. The boob just needs to dry out and then be painted black and waxed over with bronzing cream.

It was quite nice standing there, looking at it laid on the kitchen table. It makes it easier to say goodbye and I get to see it from an aspect I would otherwise never have had (mind you, I haven't tried Third Positioning my body – mmm, perhaps that's a new way of improving the getting thinner bit. More on that later.)

When Jim returned, I was just going to bed and he came and sat on the bed and we chatted about the boob and the whole experience. He's never done that before, I mean sat on the bed and chatted with me late at night, so it must have been one of those 'just right' experiences. Seemingly he knows where the boob is going to be hung, as he nodded towards the wall to my side of the bed, where we will be both be able to see it. The boob comes with hooks which we embedded in the plaster whilst making it. Jim had wondered if I could put it on a chain and wear it later! I moved the furniture in the bedroom around a few weeks back and the wall became free, odd how the mind prepares you for these things, if you let it.

I also talked about the fact that I don't know how the scar will look, and one woman I met last Tuesday said she couldn't look at her scar for months. I don't think I'll be like that; it might repulse me a bit to start. I also don't see it as 'losing my femininity'[7] either. It's good to talk. Sometimes we have to make time to talk, even it doesn't suit us. The most valuable thing you can give a person is your time.

Ah yes, on the subject of Jim, for those of you who have read *Finding The Relationship You Deserve*, you might remember our Jim is normally not the hearts-and-flowers romantic type of guy – he shows his feelings in other ways. Well it was Valentine's day on Saturday (in case you missed it). On about Weds, my traumatic day last week, I asked 'could I please have a card this year, I'm having a bad time, just one card please?' I got the card and also got a beautiful bunch of flowers. The gypsophila was all glittery and there is a 'diamond' in the centre

---

[7] One of my acquaintances (actually more than one), said she couldn't have her breast removed, as that would be
'losing her femininity'. To me my femininity is made up of many other things, how I walk, how I talk, how I express myself using words, my facial expression. I've never really felt the need to wear a bingo dress (eyes down and look in) and I'm over 50 and I've had my children. So I'd like the boob off, especially if it means I don't need to be fried by radiotherapy (how safe is that stuff?) and also it will ensure my surgeon says that the possible cancer sites are removed from that area ☺

of the rose, it came complete with vase and I was very quiet (for once). The card said 'A posy for Rosie, Jim xx!'

What else do I have to say – well Facebook is a nightmare at times, or is it some of the people on it? Let's not go there. There are some great people there. I found my Navy penfriend Keith on it, I wrote to him from when I was 16 to 18, fantastic to be in touch again.

This week I'm in Aberdeen, Diploma course at the end of the week, before that a few other things and a change to what was happening on Weds, it does mean I'm not on Facebook as it eats into my megabytes on my mobile broadband dongle.

I got this from Regan in Ellon:

'Hello again!
'If I had a list of "Things I never thought I'd read in an email" then "helped me make a plaster cast of my boob" would certainly be in there!
'I hope to see you soon Rosie. Regan xxxxx'

I noticed on Saturday one of my friends, Iain, spoke about my 'illness'. 'I'm not ill' was my reply – he looked a little pained – 'it's a dis-ease'. I've read about that principally in NLP books; I never knew what that was until Saturday, something in my body is not quite right, it's not at ease.

By the way I have visualised, and this is my visualisation, lots of little friendly spiders who have cocooned the 'little breast cancer' and contained it and there is a friendly little bee[8] inside who is busy covering the insides in beeswax to make it even safer. She's called Brenda.

I found the charger to the MP3 player on Sat and downloaded (and paid for) 'Here Comes The Sun', 'With A Little Help From My Friends', 'Good Vibrations', and 'I Will Survive' and put some other tracks on it too. Somehow Steve Andreas with his Decision Destroyer (it's an NLP technique) is bang in the middle of Stephane Grappelli, perhaps I need that in hospital too. Thanks to David T for reminding me I have an MP3 player and spurring me on to tidy my desk, I'm sure I had already tidied it! Also tidied a few other places first!

---

[8] Curiously in November 2009, I found out that bee venom is possible way of killing some tumours, and scientists are working on this. So there is something in visualisation!

NLP stuff: Visualisation

I believe there are many variations of visualisation, so here's my 'NLP Take' on it and it works, and read patiently in case you come across a bit that you find difficult, as there are ways round that.

Remember the Circle of Excellence? There is a sequence in that: See, followed by Hear, followed by Feel. That sequence is important. There is a tendency if we go to Feel first that Feel brings up negative emotions (which are just emotions, things we have created or allowed to happen to us) and those emotions mask everything else. You know that situation when you are feeling bad about something, it's often really hard to 'see clearly', 'listen carefully' etc., because the feelings get in the way.

So in the first place, have a go at seeing something. I know I mentioned spiders (I know for some people spiders are negative: was your Mum afraid of spiders? Mums generally pass on their fear of spiders – interesting thought. NLP has some good techniques to deal with this). Anyway bear with me, the spiders work for me as they are great at wrapping things up in way that it is really difficult to get out of.

So when you want to visualise, perhaps to create a Compelling Purpose to help with some healing, see that thing you want to see. For example my 'Healing Light' that I have is a gold-edged circle with translucent white in the middle that radiates out warmth, and around the edges are warming, healing rays coming to me, and they are also collecting my energy and power from the sun. I see all of that out in front of me, and build it all up, and I bring it towards me and let it envelope in particular my left breast area. I hear the sound of my voice telling me that this is healing and I'm welcoming it in and I'm feeling the healing power working around my breast and all of my lymph glands. And I do this regularly to relax and concentrate my mind on healing and peace.

With the spiders, I saw them, tiny wee things rushing around, wrapping my tumour up and creating a 'well-wrapped and protected' package that was staying put and 'Brenda' the bee was also covering this in wax, beeswax that is soft and protective and keeping me safe. The spiders were also off checking if there was anything else and if they needed to wrap that up and bring it together with the tumour. I was hearing soft 'busy' noises from the spiders and soft, comforting buzzing from Brenda and feeling calm and protected.

I still do this occasionally now, just as a check.

You can create your visualisation any way you like: remember See, Hear, Feel.

However, if you think can't See first, then start from the sense that comes to you most easily that is positive. For example, 'I can't see or visualise a tree': Okay, close your eyes, reach out in front of you, and feel the bark of the tree. What's that like? What can you feel? How does that feel? As you reach up that tree, look up, what do you see above you? When you can see that tree, open your eyes and look at it (or keep them closed, sometimes we need to close our eyes to see or visualise), what can you hear around the tree, in the tree? Should trees not work for you, what else is there that in your mind that you can touch and feel? And work from there in the same way.

All of this helps you to focus and concentrate on the good stuff that will be happening.

17th February 2009: Aberdeen

I'm in bed in the flat in Aberdeen, it's some time before 7 a.m. (I know that because the alarm has not gone off and it's after 6 a.m. because the heating is on). I feel sick – it's nine days to 'M-day' and counting – I often feel sick in the morning by the way. I reckon it's night starvation ☺ but I don't want to eat yet.

I came to Aberdeen last night – it was a good journey about 2 hours with a stop off at Morrison's. Lots of surface water just before Keith. I notice again I felt better travelling away from Forres, interesting.

My 'flatmate' isn't around, I notice he asked me when I was here this week, but didn't volunteer information on when he was here. Mmmm.

I have a client today; I wonder how they will be?

I brought my Valentine's 'posy' through with me – I seem to bring huge amounts of stuff whenever I come here, or go anywhere for that matter. In fact, I have two friends in Aberdeen who maintain 'I don't believe in travelling light!'. As a former girl guide, I just like to 'be prepared'.

I then have a couple of meetings tomorrow, Wednesday, and there's the opportunity to go to a networking event at Pittodrie (football stadium), but I also want to buy a new fridge/freezer

– a quiet one for Forres (ours keeps me awake at night with its strange noises) – and a red jacket for 19th March.

18th February 2009: Aberdeen

Perhaps it's a good thing my workshop today has been cancelled. I was really tired last evening. Maybe I am unwell? Maybe it's also because a meeting I've been arranging since last November seems to be a total mess in terms of getting the other two people to it. Maybe, just maybe I'll give up trying to get that meeting together.

I'd like to be invigorated!

I got my new red jacket yesterday, it's fab! Should I buy a fridge/freezer today or find a new hairdresser?

Later.

Mmm, I found a hairdresser – supposedly a quality one. I'm very curious about my haircut, it seems to have been chopped off pudding basin style – tomorrow will tell.

Had some curious meetings at a networking event before lunch, partially due to the fact I didn't feel too good – I didn't feel too good Tuesday/Wednesday but that might have been the all-new Vegan diet I took on inadvertently (with hindsight). Felt better after a tuna jacket potato once I'd persuaded Café Coast 'No, I do not need cheese on it'. Why do the Scots like cheese on everything (almost)? Why do they really do healthy eating badly?

And do I think I'm ill, because some people keep on telling me I am?

Also having problems sending emails – is it the dongle or Windows Vista [turned out it was the thick granite walls on the house in Aberdeen, a common problem with mobile signals and WiFi seemingly?]

I am concocting a wondrous tea of falafel, tomatoes and spinach – I quite fancy beef burger and chips, or one of my flatmate's pork pies (from the fridge, perhaps not!).

19th February 2009: Aberdeen

Thursday – Aberdeen Winter Diploma day 3 – another interesting day ahead – I always love to find out what people have in store for themselves.

Feel better this morning – eating better – perhaps the sugar overdose (note to self, be 100% certain on amounts of sugar in so-called healthy cereal bars).

My hair looks a little better in the mirror this morning – be interested to see it after washing and blow drying it. It's a bit short at the back.

Oh yes, my tea was good last night.

21st February 2009: The conservatory diary extract

Well, it's different as a topic! Over the last few days, conservatories have come up as a topic on my NLP Diploma course. I notice, in fact, conservatories are a recurring theme on Practitioner/Diploma courses. To be honest, guys – why? Most people seem to have hassle/can't get started etc. with building their conservatory, and personally our conservatory is a huge waste of space. Why? Well, it's taken away part of the garden. Gardens are places for children to play in and grannies! We also have shrubs in our garden; somehow the idea of the English lawn on which you can sit out and have tea gets missed by some of the Scots (well one in particular)! Never mind. I will never be mowing this lawn round the damn shrubs (aka odd bushes which serve no purpose in my mind).

Currently our conservatory houses a king-size mattress, anyone fancy one? Why? Well, last night we slept in our all-new lambs wool bedding, in fact Jim must still be enjoying it as he hasn't risen and I want to have a luxurious Lush bath (have got two different bath bombs to find the one I want for this coming Thursday morning), but I am waiting for Jim to get up as he has a routine in the morning! Until yesterday, the conservatory housed the dishwasher (aka threat to Jim's manhood – long story but he likes to wash the dishes?!). I finally deduced that was why the dishwasher was not being installed so we sold it, to the benefit of my daughter whose dishwasher it was; it was only a wee one.

Our conservatory also houses the 1970s walnut (broken top) 'pimp's' (Kristin's words) cocktail cabinet that I ousted from the sitting room and I live in hope that it will leave the house. Currently it acts as storage for Leon and Nico's toys that are also a feature of the conservatory, the odd wooden crane and bulldozer, along with hand puppets (ah, they're Granny's actually) and a few other things. Plus some items Rosie will eBay one day and the TV Jim watches either (a) when Rosie is firmly ensconced with her ten cushions on the couch in the sitting room or (b) when he thinks I don't know he's in there watching sport during the day with the sound turned down – the self-employed don't like people skiving watching TV during the day, especially those who lie about being retired ☺

Our conservatory is really a bit like a greenhouse, a place for drying the washing and glorified storage area. Why? Cos it hasn't got a proper roof on it! So you can't use it as a spare bedroom, dining room or useful place either in the bad weather cos it's cold or the good weather cos it's too hot (rarely where we live ☺).

Anyway. I'm fine, I was in Aberdeen most of the week and did drive back last night as I felt okay and wanted to come home (so I can sit at the PC at 8 a.m. in the morning writing my diary ☺). And I did meet some really important people in Aberdeen as I predicted on my Facebook account.

I hoped last night my 'lump' had gone, the swelling from the invasion of the 'fine' needle used for the biopsy has gone down. I can tell you, no one, but no one who really believes that it is a 'fine' needle, and it will not hurt and all you will feel is the pressure, has ever had a flaming 'fine needle biopsy' taken, but you are in a state of shock so that a red hot poker up the bum wouldn't hurt (well not at the time). The bruising is almost gone thanks to my comfrey salve (haven't gone for the castor oil job again ☺). Ah well, that'll soon change.

I realise that 26th February is quite a significant date for me – for those of you who don't yet know I have quite a phenomenal memory (especially if you owe me money ☺). 26th February 2004 was a Thursday and it had been snowing, certainly in Nairn where I lived at the time, it was a night to remember in my life (apart from, on leaving the house, a phone call from Kristin to tell me she was splitting with Leon's dad [that's a book in itself – Nico's dad too and Nico wasn't even around then]). I was most sublimely seduced – things like that stay etched on a woman's memory – it was a wonderful evening, involving a piano amongst other things ☺. I'll write about it in my memoirs (or sooner – when I get on *Loose Women* maybe).

26th February 2008 was a significant date in Jim's life, because he went on a huge ferry for the first time in his life from Rosyth to Zeebrugge, and subsequently experienced Belgium, a bit of Holland and Germany all on the wrong side of the road, in the passenger seat of my car, and Rosie in a bad temper when she has missed the turning. We went to my friend Emmi's ninetieth birthday party, a very significant lady in my life! She's the mother of my friend Margit, we have been friends since we were 16 and without her and her family I would never have gone to live in Germany and never have had my children and thus Leon and Nico would not be around.

So this year it's Raigmore Hospital, Inverness on 26th February – yippee.

I have had lots of hugs and good wishes this week and Liz in Glenshiel has sent me some really nice soap! I have also been given a book of angels with fantastic illustrations. It was passed on to me, so I'm aiming to pass it on very soon ☺. Thank you everyone.

And my brother has written to me – this is a surreal experience (and would be another book) but I'm quite tickled by it.

'Hi Sis,

'Thought you might like to see some pics of the view from where we are staying. It's up on the top of a hill overlooking the harbor so we get a sea view to the front and the back. Not only that but being so high it's nice and breezy so wonder of wonders – no mossies. Cannot remember coming to this part of the world and not applying mossie spray! Bit wet and windy – it's blowing Roman Abramavitch's mega yacht all over the harbor, ugly bloody thing – -like a cross between a Russian warship and floating fish factory ship – it's that big blue and white thing top left in the harbor pic – it has a 65 foot sailing boat on the back together with a 50 foot speed boat so you can imagine how big it is. You can't see the submarine because he keeps that inside. Roman, I'll take the boat but you can keep the football team.

'Still, for £125 a week this place is pretty good value although you need a car too as its well off the beaten track – £75 a week for a broken down, oil leaking, open sided ex-Barbados hire car – known locally as a tourist egg box because it looks a bit like an egg box I suppose. Or maybe it's a reference to the young chickens inside the car – I dunno but for £200 a week plus food, Bobs your mother's brothers as far as I am concerned. And god bless the internet for allowing me to work from here as well. Beats sitting in an office in London and having to be nice to people. Plus I spend at least sixty per cent of my time in the office behind the computer anyway.

'Keep yer peckah up kid.'

He's my 'little brother', I have written to tell him I learned to 'go on holiday' 2 years ago, which involves no Internet or phones. Bequia is in the Caribbean for the unknowing – he has been retiring out there since he was 40; he just turned 54 this month. There's a significant seven word phrase in that message

– tells you a lot about my little bro ☺ My mother says the real brother was not abducted by aliens as I sometimes think.

Jim's up at last; perhaps I get in my bath soon then!

Boob (plaster cast one, I hasten to add) will be painted this weekend, I sawed and sanded the edges before I left for Aberdeen on Monday, some bits broke off. Now thanks in part to my Dad who used to make plaster casts of people's stumps (as in legs, he was a prosthesetist and also the number of times I have broken arms and legs in my life – it was the gin my mother put in the milk – she will go mad about that!). I know how to use a plaster bandage – my Dad used to bring home little green tins of the stuff – what did we use those for? I was able to repair the bits (round the outside) of my plaster cast) and it's all nice and dry now so painting will commence and then hanging on the wall ☺.

I also have to complete my insurance claim form, for the cancelled holiday at Easter and Jim will be taking it to the GPs. I have received a treacly letter from the surgery and a rubbish letter from the NHS who seem to have missed part of my complaint completely; I'll save it all until later.

By the way if you want to ask me anything do, my friend Sam W (there are two Sams receiving this letter) asked me was it okay to ask a question – yes I'll answer to the best of ability.

Hell we really need to share this more – there is NO absolutely NO shame in having cancer and certainly not in having the boob off, my femininity will remain. You can look at the scar after if you like (well I draw the line at guys) and Jo's already asked to touch the false one (the prosthesis I will receive – well my Dad has a prosthesis and I hope to hell they give me the right one, cos I tell you an extra leg will not fit down my bra!!)

Have great weekend.

23 February 2009: My sister

I phoned my sister, did you know I have a sister? I have another mother too.[9] They both live in Germany – it's another long story. Emmi, I mentioned her last time is my other my mother (my Mum knows) and her daughter Margit is like a sister to me. I spent a lot of time deciding how I tell Margit, do I tell her? (And after my son's reaction and that of another person – there seem to be 'wrong ways'. Scuse me no one checked the 'right way' with me!! I just was told 'but we know it's not a cyst – it's a little breast cancer'. That's one of those occasions when in a way life slows down whilst you process that fact – and although you know you've heard it, somehow you haven't, and that's probably cos you don't want it to be true, well not for you, for that someone else in that parallel universe. It's not happening to me! And then reality strikes – 'shit it is me! In my case – shit I'd better deal with it.

A tip – avoid these questions: 'Why me?' (there's no answer to that one), 'I've had most things in life happen to me, there can't be anything else can there? (oh yes there can!),[10] 'Can't it happen to someone else?' (well it probably can but then that

---

[9] Sadly, Emmi Herbert died in August 2009 during the writing of this book. She is much missed but she had lived to a ripe old age and experienced many things in her life.

[10] If you don't know about some of the other things, read my book *Finding the Relationship You Deserve.*

interesting holiday – I seem to remember that was immedia\
after Kristin did her disappearing act. She upped and left hom\
at 17 for about a week, something to do with 'me not needing
her any more' now that Michael was there and 'her father and
the fact that I had never said anything good or bad about him'.
Also about the time Michael started to behave oddly. You know
my life might have been so much simpler had I not gone to
Germany and actually met my Navy penfriend then (but we'll
never know, will we Keith?).

Anyway I phoned Margit, her first reaction as 'Oh Gott'. Well
her sister in law died of lung cancer last year, and then I said
immediately but I'm living until 97, she said she hoped a lot
longer, we're the same age; well she's 6 weeks older. We have
known one another since we were 16 and have been through a
\t together and separately. She sighed and said (in German of
\urse) 'you know this year I really thought things are going so
\ll for you.' Yes me too ☺

\ink this new book might be called 'Hear that it's Cancer –
\ the Person and talk to them about them'. Must find
\ething snappier ☺

\ouse smells very nice, the bathroom is full of various Lush
\omb smells, it'll be the purple one on Thursday I think.
\orning it's going to be rushing round with the hair
\g cream on for 10 mins, for those of you who make

would be unfair for them too). Actually the 'Why me' one – I think it's anthroposophy that says we choose our lives, well we have a kind of choice, or we see our lives at the time of th[e] birth, and yes I know Wordsworth:

Our birth is but a sleep and a forgetting:
The Soul that rises with us, our life's star,
Hath had elsewhere its setting,
And cometh from afar:
Not in entire forgetfulness,
And not in utter nakedness,
But trailing clouds of glory do we come
From God, who is our home

*William Wordsworth, 'Intimations of Immortality f[rom]
Recollections of Early Childhood'*

Was I on something at the time of my birth [in a previous?] life? Mother, were you on drugs, or was [this]? There's also something about in this life [and a?] previous life and we were probably the oth[er's?] life.[11] Well, when I get my time machine [I'll go] back in time and have words with the[m]. Perhaps use some NLP on them!

I went to the Lake District for my for[ty...] (there's a poem called Michael by [Wordsworth]

---

11 This is esoteric science, from Rudol[f]

pictures in your heads, please switch off visual capabilities – as I have to do this naked – women will know what I mean! The office smells of geranium and clary sage, part of yesterday's calming procedure.

I felt sick yesterday morning, sick at the thought of Thursday and the unknown and who knows what, hey it's my head. I can create my own sick feelings very well! Have a new Circle of Excellence, lying down and boy can I do deep breathing! Ah well.

I also received this, this morning, for those of you in the know, my Practitioner and Diploma participants have to write reflections on what they learned at the weekend or over the last session they spent with us. This from Sara G:

'When reflecting on the weekend, I can't not mention the news you shared with us. I'm not going to linger too much on that, as I suspect you would prefer to read about something else – I just want to say thank-you for sharing it in a way that helped maintain a good and useful state for me that weekend. I have thought a lot about the conversation that came out of this over the weekend and the way in which the words we use can have so much influence on our state of health and mind. I shared my Dad's experience of doctors telling him he would never be well again – he took these words very much as a challenge and was determined to prove the doctor wrong. He is now much improved, he refers quite frequently to the words the doctor used about him 'never being well again' – these words are significant to him and I think played a fundamental part in his recovery. Since the weekend I've also reflected on my Mum who has also been ill in the past, with what now appears to have been food allergies (wheat). When thinking about her, I can see now that she actually needed a health professional to tell her there was something wrong before she would do anything about it. Doctors were actually telling her there was nothing wrong with her, which she found infuriating. I suspected wheat intolerance and got her several books on how to deal with it. She wouldn't do anything however until she saw a kinesiologist and he diagnosed wheat intolerance. She then got herself better, principally by changing her diet – but for her to embark on that first step required a health professional to tell her that something was wrong. Such a different need and reaction to words . . .'

Mmm, bloomin words and bloomin doctors – probably my greatest worries for the coming time – ah well strong stuff this NLP. Mind you this also came on Saturday:

'Rosie, so nice to hear from you albeit with sad news. Knowing your grit, determination and positive attitude, I am confident you will be back in the swing of things in no time! I don't 'ride off into the sunset' until June so, hopefully, we'll be able to 'connect' before then. My very best wishes. George.'

Today I have Pilates, back in my usual class with the groaning minnies – I mean that nicely – and the wonderful Sara Hunt,[12] the woman who knows my body is out of sync by 2 mm, the woman who will help me stretch my way back to fitness. Then off to Aberdeen, again later for a presentation tomorrow to Aberdeen Businesswomen, 'Influencing with Integrity' – there's

---

[12] I recommend 'Body Control Pilates' – I have experience of several kinds of Pilates and Pilates teachers and the 'Body Control Pilates' teachers look at you as an individual within a group –, well Sara Hunt (www.pilatesinverness.com) does ☺ If you can't do something, it probably is because your body is a different shape.

no such thing as a free lunch ☺. Tomorrow evening, *Fame* the musical with Fiona S, Sara G and Susan (who has hopefully had a good time with her friend in Stirling who had gone into hiding after her mastectomy). Then Wednesday, the day with a client before I come back home ☺

I mentioned earlier had my hair cut in Aberdeen last week, I am not quite sure if I would recommend them, it was not the most interesting haircut I have ever had, mind you perhaps telling the hairdresser why I was going in hospital was not a good idea (note to self).

Leon arranged to visit yesterday; well I told Leon I had a plane and a helicopter (Lego from a charity shop). After Nico got over his usual sulk (about something someone did that didn't suit him, but we don't know what it was), both boys fought over the plane, the helicopter and the plane, and the helicopter, not necessarily in that order. Mummy removed the plane, and Nico finally washed all the ducks in the bathroom hand basin, they will have great complexions as they appear to have been washed in my face mask! (Plastic ducks I may add – mine, thirteen of them – I once had 100 – excellent for counting in German in case you wondered!). So ultimately they ate my freshly baked loaf of bread with great gusto (who was gusto, anyone know?).

I have written to my usual hairdresser, Clare, to ask for forgiveness and when will she be back at work, let's hope the salon passes the letter on. [They didn't until she actually came back to work ☹]

A face just appeared at the door enquiring why I was up and would I like to come back to bed? He was sleeping earlier and wouldn't give me a hug, so short of beating him up and asking for the hug, I'll get up. So I'll leave this for now.

One more to come this week before my date with the surgeon.

I'm goin' to live forever

Death and dying. If you think for one moment I didn't think about dying, you are so wrong. Probably right at the very onset of this experience, my mind might temporarily have gone to dying. I'm not conscious of that, I suspect I might have done. As a teenager with my teenage angst, I sometimes thought about dying. A bit melodramatic, on my deathbed with everyone around me, teachers, friends, family, all regretting the terrible things they had ever done to me ☺ Or Ophelia floating down the stream ☺ Certainly just before I upped and offed from my first marriage I did once contemplate what life might be like without me and decide really that wasn't a successful outcome for my then very small children and did I want to leave them with the violent alcoholic of a man? So I might have temporarily flashed off in my mind to life without me. But I think it was more than likely as nowadays, that what I did was I looked for and added the sounds and got good feelings about how life would be with me still around.

A couple of things I do know I did, shortly before I went into hospital. I asked Jim to get me the metal box down out of the cupboard, in which we keep our important documents, because I said I want to check my funeral arrangements. He looked at me quizzically and asked 'Was you planning on dying?' No I just wanted to check. I wrote my funeral arrangements (now I have to live in hope that they will be carried out, after all when I'm gone my family can do what they like really, I can't get back to stop them). I wrote down my order of service for my funeral in 1995, that was the year after my second husband died and I realised even though we had talked about death and dying, I had no idea what he wanted said, sung or played at this funeral service and with hindsight I would have done it differently (played 'The Final Countdown', a track that Michael blasted out on many a Sunday morning through the patio doors in Linthorpe, Middlesbrough) but I was too distraught at the time.

So mine is:

For my funeral

Music to enter by – Pachelbel's 'Canon' played by the Hallé Orchestra (it must be the Hallé Orchestra).

Reading – Robert Frost's 'The Road not Taken'. (My Mum gave a poetry book several years ago, *Poem for the Day*. For the 30th September, my birthday, the poem is 'The Road Not Taken'. My Mum dedicates that poem to me, she says it is about me – read it).

Music – John Denver's 'Annie's Song' (I might change this now)

Then a speech by someone who knows me. (Well, most probably my daughter Kristin or Susan Raeper, as I'm assuming I will outlive my Mum and the other two know me pretty well, well they are two of the very few people who are never surprised by anything I say I will do, or have done ☺).

Reading – Christina Rosetti's 'Song'

Music – John Denver's 'Follow Me'

Music to leave by – 'I've Had the Time of My Life' from *Dirty Dancing*

Believe me whatever happened in my life, basically I enjoyed, and I respected and appreciated the people I met, even if they then let themselves down and were disappointed.

Often times in NLP and I'm sure in other disciplines, there is the suggestion that we write our own obituary and then work towards living that. Perhaps just reading some of the testimonials I have received is enough of an obituary?

Another thing, I've mentioned Terry Pratchett before, remember? Now I like Terry Pratchett's *Discworld* series, the character Death (tall guy in a long black cloak with a scythe) often appears and when he does he speaks in capital letters! And why not?

One day not long before my op, I was in the garden hanging out the washing and for some reason 'Four and twenty blackbirds' came into my head. You know it, do you? 'The maid was in the garden hanging out the clothes, when down came a blackbird etc.' And then for some reason in my wild imagination, I saw and heard, 'GOOD MORNING.' Oops no time to wonder if I had completely lost it. 'Err well, am I going to d . . .?'. 'NO JUST POPPED IN TO SAY HELLO AND IT'S NOT YOUR TIME YET.' Thanks Terry Pratchett ☺

You can tell me anything you like about that experience. I think it was just my imagination and my subconscious/unconscious processing something, perhaps my will to live (after all there are many well-documented cases of people who believe they will die and just do that) and boy do I have a will to live.

I just thought I'd mention all this stuff, in case anyone reading this might think, disgustingly positive people, never think about death and dying (in fact perhaps because we do and we dismiss it as not happening, yet, or it not being the right time, then in as much as we have a degree of control over this living, we will continue to live for a while longer). And also I've experienced that we deal with death badly, in as much as we don't talk about it, or if we do, we do it in a small voice in very hushed tones and a small voice, like this font here, and we leave people 'to get on with it' and that's often getting on with it in a very unuseful way, in my experience. Unuseful for the individual let alone anyone else, but that's another story.

25th February 2009: Keeping you abreast of the situation

Well, it's Wednesday, which as you know comes before Thursday, it's 22.30 and I was going to bed, I was also trying to work out how to get all of the addresses I send this email to out of the locked file and into my Yahoo account in an easy manner, ah easy, and Microsoft not compatible.

I hear lights being switched on or off and I take it that's my call to go to bed. Might come back in the morning.

. . .

Now it's Thursday, guess what? I got up early, well I was awake. Sara Kennedy is not on the radio at this time in the morning, it's Richard Allison (this will only mean something to you if you listen to Radio 2 – ever).

I need to have words with the butler, he has not posted my post (from Monday) – he hides things in piles (no comments). I ordered Jim a chauffeur's hat on Monday on eBay, he had said he couldn't chauffer me over the next few weeks without a hat!

On Monday as I got ready to leave Forres for Aberdeen I wondered why I was 'messing about' and not leaving, so in my best NLP fashion I did a bit of wondering/wandering in my subconscious and noticed I didn't want to leave because when I came back, today (as in Thursday 26th February 2009 'Mastectomy' day) would be very close. Anyway I did leave and got to Aberdeen in good time, good journey and unpacked my stuff and the rest of the stuff for Rebecca for my Practitioner course weekend in March (only just around the corner).

My presentation for Aberdeen Businesswomen on Tuesday went well, with lots of state maintenance.

Fame was fantastic, Fiona S picked me up and we had an interesting drive to HMT in Aberdeen, note to NLP trainers everywhere, if you want to find out more about how your course participants process, let them drive you somewhere. The drive was also a fantastic experience as well, thanks Fiona.

The cast of *Fame* put their heart and soul into the performance, at the interval I spied my friend Sam G, madly waving from the upper circle, she tells me her husband possibly knows my surgeon, do I get better treatment that way? At the end we all got the opportunity to stand up and belt out 'I'm goin live for ever' yeh! I bought a *Fame* wristband: when they tell me later today to get ready for theatre, will I be able to wear it? (Think about that last sentence).

We also had an interesting conversation about knickers. I have to wear all cotton underwear in the operating theatre (will I cause sparks?). Sara G wanted to know 'how will they know?', 'will they look?', well you know I'll be out for the count so how will I know? And do you know how difficult it is to find all cotton knickers, mine are 98%, as 2% of the trim is not cotton, very complex. Best big, sensible white knickers from Markies. Good side is if you want to know how old I am – it will be 18. (You know the joke – little girl asks grandma 'how old are you?', grandma says 'I don't know dear', little girl says 'look in the back of your knickers the label will tell you'. Whey hey.)[13]

Mmm, at this point it is 6 a.m., the former president of RBS is receiving how much as a pension? Why didn't I stay in banking?

In years to come, will this book become part of the English curriculum at school? There's a thought.

Yesterday I spent all day with a client – great stuff, we started out with so much detail and got it down to about four steps she needed to take – Mapping Out Your Life – literally in some ways in her case – I love this stuff.

---

[13] I discovered in hospital and after my op about the knickers. As another patient on the ward was going to theatre for an op that would have been around the knicker covering area, the nurse asked the question as to the cotton content of her knickers. Another patient asked why and the explanation given was that if the surgeon needs to cauterise or some such, non-cotton knickers might fuse with the skin – ouch!

Then I drove back from Aberdeen and had four long phone calls, my Mum, Rebecca who was on top form (as so often), seems to be 'sharing her screen' with some guy in India, the result of too much of this she says is that you may have to go the 'VD-U Clinic', Alison (middle 'daughter-in-law') and Fiona (eldest 'daughter-in-law'). Took a while to prise the phone off Jim, as Fiona does not phone often (Ally phones every week) and Fiona was really phoning to speak to me – he found that hard to understand – hmm. In-between, a lovely text message from my daughter and a message from her on Facebook. Fortunately during the first two calls I was 'hands free' and was able to unpack my stuff and do various bits and pieces, my intention was to catch up on things.

My best news yesterday was that I can have breakfast this morning, not as the letter from the hospital said 'nothing to eat after midnight' last night, as the op is not until 1.30 p.m. I might fall over.

The bronzed boob is on the wall. I have a photo, it's funny, I'd be quite happy to put it in the book [sorry folks, not doing illustrations this time ☺], but not share it yet, maybe that's because we are still so closely connected?

I've been studying the area underneath my eyes recently, there is a marked 'tired line' – I put on extra amounts of 'Protect and Perfect' last night! But I'm looking out for 'the Savage bags'.

Now if, 'like me' you read Terry Pratchett, this is not some form of wildly angry luggage, but 'bags under my eyes', my Dad's family have 'bags under their eyes', my mother has often in the past maintained my brother and I would get them too. My eyes are looking very dark underneath; this could of course be a result of lack of sleep!

The hospital is in for a treat later today – during the pre-op stuff when I was asked 'any adverse reaction to anaesthetics' I carefully missed out the 'yes I get hyper' and 'if you give me painkillers, I turn into something like what I can only assume is Rosie on LSD' (never having tried any kind of recreational drug and I am proud of that fact, I wouldn't know – I saw earlier a heading in health supplement catalogue 'Love your joints'(to my little brother this would have a different meaning to the one intended ☺) – I digress. My mother has witnessed this phenomenon, Rosie hyper. I mentioned it to Rebecca, she commented yes sometimes hospitals miss the administration of doses according to personality, instead of things like height and weight. So they will slap me with lots cos as you know I am undertall for my weight, and being the extrovert I am (often but not always as my Myers-Briggs personality type indicator indicates – some of you will know what that means), I'll be bouncing off the walls tonight. Hee hee.

Must away for light breakfast. And then bath with Lush bath bomb and then, well I don't really know. I have to give myself into 'other people's hands'!

Bye for now – I'll be back. (And there's a few tears in my eyes, either that or it's raining?)

2nd March 2009: Not lobster pots then?

I couldn't resist that title, and you will be wondering, what is she on now?

Outside the day room at the hospital, where it was good to go to use my mobile phone, there were often two oystercatchers. Now I love these birds with their long red beaks and distinctive black and white colouring and the fact that you will nearly always see them in pairs. This was always the same pair. How does she know that, the damn things look the same? Well one had a lump of grass stuck to one foot, I assume it had stood in something noxious and sticky and then either hopped on the grass and got grass stuck to it, or perhaps the sticky stuff already had grass on it. This stuck lump was like a very awkward clown's boot and the oystercatcher just carried on being an oystercatcher, as animals and birds do, ok a bit broke, fell off, and something attached itself to me. I'll get on with it! A little like me I thought and I also remembered a conversation I had quite a few years ago with my daughter Kristin.

I was living in Latheron (17 miles south of Wick in Caithness) and Kristin was up to stay, we drove up to Dunnet Head, Dunnet Head is actually the most northerly tip of the British Isles, not John O'Groats. On the way up there, there is an old watermill and we stopped off there to look at the mill and the mill pond and I told Kristin of a time I had previously been up there, with my friends Jon and Brenda and there were two oystercatchers running up and down on the roof of the mill, presumably to distract us from their clutch of eggs. 'Oh', Kristin said, seemingly unimpressed (this is the girl who as a teenager went bird watching on the Farne Isles with school). We got in the car and as we drove further on towards Dunnet Head, suddenly she burst out laughing, 'Ah, Oystercatchers are birds, not like lobster pots then?' The birds reminded me of a sunny day spent with my daughter BG (before grandsons).

3rd March 2009: Reshaping my life

Hey it's 5.26 a.m., I know that without looking at the clock because the train for Edinburgh is just leaving Forres station, in the quiet of the morning I can hear that. I caught it once last year to go to somewhere in the depths of Oxfordshire (I think) to speak at a conference on emissions for the nuclear industry! (That's another story involving the words 'risk' and 'discharge').

Well I'm home – let's start with last Thursday 26th February 2009.

So we left home at 7.30 a.m. approx and drove to Inverness, on the way whilst I'm starting to worry and wonder how I 'should be' feeling, I looked across at Jim, my man was turning decidedly grey and looking very odd. 'Are you ok?' I asked. Yes he gruffed back, 'not awake yet, middle of the night.' Mmm, from my viewpoint, this looked like a Jim who was going to get very upset. Was just about to text his middle daughter Jean, when I discovered a text from her 'Thinking of you.' I texted back thanks and asked her something along the lines of your Dad not looking good (to me) – 'please look after this bear'. (The bear is a very important metaphor to me in respect of Jim, very huggy). Jean asked, rightly does he have his mobile and is it switched on? Always justified, the mobile aspect of a mobile phone is not one Jim always understands and sometimes just the phone being in the car is mobile ☺. He did have phone.

We got to Ward 8 at Raigmore at 8.30 a.m., it looked a very quiet place. A man (doctor I discovered later) told us to ring the small hand bell on the desk, and from nowhere a bright and sparkly staff nurse called Eilidh Begg (from Wick nonetheless) appeared 'you're coming to me' she said brightly – ah expected, and I did feel welcomed. Later in the day she may have regretted meeting me, bet she was glad to go home that day ☺ The 'ladies' on the ward were having their breakfast, so Jim had to sit in the day room (quite why you need privacy to eat, I am not sure). I was admitted (several times that day I was asked the same questions, I'm either to believe no one had asked these questions before or they were just checking did I remember what I said?) I was visited by a young woman aged about 17 in a Ra Ra skirt and opaque blue tights with lots of hair who told me she was 'Tory a doctor'. Who was I to argue, we were after all in a hospital and she had a clipboard and a lanyard round her neck. Mind you I noticed the lanyards vary and I am getting older?

Eilidh gave me a fetching gown and some even more fetching white stockings and nifty little injection to 'thin my blood' which, as she said, didn't hurt (she was the only one who gave said injection from whom it didn't hurt). After 9 a.m. I sent Jim away and I 'settled in'. There were six of us on the six-bed ward at that time, one of whom had had a mastectomy on the

Tuesday, so I was able to speak to her about how she was doing. She was doing well.

I was also able to get on Facebook from the 'station' next to my bed, seems I wore it out later, as I couldn't get back on.

Then some waiting and some more waiting, I was told I would get my pre-med about 12.30. About 12.30 lunch appeared, not for me, and almost at the same time my consultant appeared with junior surgeon in tow. We had the most fascinating time, probably not if you were having your lunch on the other side of the curtain ☺ They drew on me with a felt tip marker – all those times you spend telling your children not to do that, first a big arrow pointing to the left, very useful really to be honest I thought, an error doesn't bear thinking about.

A long discussion ensued between junior surgeon (in green scrubs) and my consultant (aka to other patients in the ward 'serious eye candy', not my type – too easy for me to embarrass ☺). Mr D frequently asked if I was ok with this discussion – it was the most interesting thing that happened to me on the day seriously, yes I reassured him. Then I remembered to ask him if he knew Alan G from Aberdeen, the junior surgeon who had been at Raigmore last year. Oh yes, well his wife is a friend of mine. At which point Mr D pointed out to junior doctor (Mhairi) who Alan is, she reckons she's a friend of Sam's too, might be her head somersaulted at the time, I am old enough to be Sam's Mum, in fact Sam's about 10 months younger than Kristin (age of no relevance to me, where my friends are concerned, it's the quality ☺). The discussion over the incisions continued. At one point Mr D told Mhairi they would be 'cutting a flap' as you would for a below the knee amputation. 'I know exactly what you mean,' I said. He looked at me in that (a) ah yes, patient can hear what I'm saying, and (b) oops – patient replied 'my Dad has a below the knee amputation, I know exactly what you mean!'

Both doctors then chatted to me with my gown on and said the anaesthetist would be down to see me shortly. On cue, he appeared through the curtain. Fantastic. Anaesthetist was horrified at the thought of my crowns (on my teeth) and I warned him my dentist is in Wick! He also asked whether I have any reaction to anaesthetics. 'Yes,' I replied, 'I go a bit hyper afterwards.' 'Oh,' he said, 'that'll be fun in the recovery room.' Mr D looked at me and said 'I think she means we'll be coping with it on the ward!' Too right.

'Well,' said Mr D, 'they'll be down for you soon,' and on opening the curtains – on cue again – my chariot awaited ☺ 'We'd better hurry,' said the departing consultant, who also helped me get out of bed and asked had I been listening to my relaxation CD on the MP3 player. 'No', I replied, 'Dire Straits!'

So off I went. The pre-op area is like a huge barn in Raigmore, two people were already waiting on their chariots and another lady appeared after I was wheeled into my bay. No time to think as I breathed into my recumbent circle of excellence, I was wheeled through to my anaesthetic room. The anaesthetist was mumbling about my crowns and stuck a cannula in the back of my right hand and the next thing I knew was, someone was waking me up from one of those dreams you're enjoying (and I have no idea what it was) and I then was wheeled back to the ward. Eilidh was insistent I wear an oxygen mask; I felt as if I'd OD'd on entinox and kept on taking the mask off. Seemingly I'd been in respiratory distress (to my way of thinking if anyone cuts your natural air supply for a few hours you'd be distressed), must have been trying to do slow relaxed breathing, contrary to their wishes seemingly! Also I was dehydrated, well guys I drink lots of water in a day and hadn't had a drink since sloshing my foul-tasting mouthwash round my mouth earlier in the day.

I had to stop writing due to overuse of left hand, it makes bits jangle at the nerve endings where the five (yes just five ☺) lymph glands were removed: five is good, five is one more than my prognosis. So I'm just using the right hand. Typing is good as I am sitting in the kneeling chair, as my back aches from lying down too long. This is the second night I slept really well, believe me really well, it is not perhaps how I would like it to be as turning to the left is no go, but it is really well.

On 26th February in the evening Jim came to see me and I got a message Kristin had rung, for those of you who don't know I was on Facebook at some point after the op. I also watched *Loose Women* at about 2.30 in the morning ☺

Hospital is very tiring. People wake you up, people moan and groan, and on our ward they talked a lot, disturbing my reading and then it seems there's this never-ending eating. You've just had one meal and they bring you another one. Or some people seem to get streams of chocolates and biscuits (I'd asked for fruit only). Healthy eating is seemingly a concept in the NHS – it hasn't quite made it on to the menus or the plates. My consultant told me on Friday I could go home on Monday ☺ Jean came to visit me after lunch and brought me lots of books. Then Rebecca came with soya milk and an Alexander McCall Smith book, I can't quite get Alexander McCall Smith! She also brought *Positive Thinking for Calvinists* – fantastic book. Sandra R also came to visit, she's a lovely positive lady who has popped up in my life over the past 4 years ☺ After that, one would hope one could rest – no chance. More talking, visit by the physio who missed me the day before? I don't know when she came, unless it was during my theatre visit (and this is the only time I saw a physio). Then food. Jim visited and brought me Connie Fisher's new CD – on the Monday as I drove to Pilates I heard Connie speaking on Radio 4 and then a snippet of this was played. When I embarked on my brief singing career from 2002–2004, this was the first song I learned. I realise I have this outcome, so the words of songs can also shape our lives:

There's a saying old, says that love is blind
Still we're often told, seek and ye shall find
So I'm going to seek a certain lad I've had in mind

Looking everywhere, haven't found him yet
He's the big affair I cannot forget
Only man I ever think of with regret

I'd like to add his initial to my monogram
Tell me, where is the shepherd for this lost lamb?

There's a somebody I'm longin to see
I hope that he, turns out to be
Someone who'll watch over me

I'm a little lamb who's lost in the wood
I know I could, always be good
To one who'll watch over me

Although he may not be the man some
Girls think of as handsome
To my heart he carries the key

Won't you tell him please to put on some speed

Follow my lead, oh, how I need

Someone to watch over me.

George Gershwin, 'Someone to watch over me'

He found me. Curious ☺

8th March 2009: Softees

The Saturday morning in hospital when my consultant arrived, I was wandering around the bed, reapportioning all my books. He asked me what I was doing. 'Trying to escape?' I replied hopefully. 'You can go home tomorrow,' he said, 'we'll see you in clinic.' Yeh hey.

Sat afternoon I waited patiently for my visitors in the ward, in the end I walked to the hospital entrance and waited by the café. Here I am waiting for the most important person in my life. From sometime after Michael's death in 1994 on and off until 2002 when I moved from Caithness down to Nairn and a little while after that I had this thing called depression, on and off. I dislike the word depression it means so many things to many people and it can be caused by so many things, and it was possibly unresolved grief at that time [now sorted since using NLP and with thanks to a colleague of mine, Andy Hunt]. Anyway I digress. On 31st December 2003, the person who enabled me to make life worth living (for me) was born, and I am very lucky that on that afternoon whilst visiting my parents in Hertfordshire, not long after being back from Christmas in Frankfurt, that I had a text message from Kristin saying 'your grandson would like to see you'. So I met Leon Michael when he was around 3 hours old and beautiful and smiling (since then he can scowl, and how). Because it was New Year's Eve and Homerton Hospital (Hackney, London) I was left with Kristin and Leon for a long time and at least able to explain, yes breastfeeding is not easy you're both new to this game and need to practice ☺ That night I floated back to my brother's flat on air and exhilaration. In later times Leon's smiley face has been around when I was going through a difficult time, suddenly moving house from Nairn to Forres, his utter joy at meeting his brother (this may have changed since) and many other occasions. Thursday this week when he was with us for the day because he had tummy ache and he talked and talked and talked, I may have temporarily revised my opinion ☺ and he sulked because he couldn't have his own way.

However last Saturday I was waiting for them all (Kristin, Jim, Leon and Nico) and I was able to walk back to the ward holding hands with Leon and Nico. I asked Leon if he remembered the last time we held hands walking in a hospital. 'To see Mummy and Nico?' he replied. (Nico was even younger than Leon when I first met him and still in the delivery room with Mummy and that was where we decided on his name).

Chaos ensued in our room on Ward 8, in spite of us just being three patients left, so we adjourned to the café and fed the small boys (including Jim).

In the evening I was reading in peace and not expecting visitors when Jean arrived with Alasdair and the more beautiful every time I see her. Abigail, legs and hair to die for and only 13. A great honour, these visitors.

On Saturday evening, the staff nurse for the night (surname Cavell nonetheless) showed me softees[14] not to be confused with softies (a variety of bread roll locally), bras with pockets and a couple of samples of prostheses (breast forms, 'chicken fillets'), which I could touch and hold. The softee I would get next day, and the prosthesis will be measured etc. in clinic. My appointment with the consultant is Friday 13th – must be good.

Sunday was escape day, my all-time favourite nurse on Ward 8 was Kirsteen Williamson (I won't mention that she left me attached to the blood pressure monitor during visiting time on Sat – I just took it off and left ☺). Kirsteen removed the drain which takes away blood and the lymph (when the lymph fluid starts to appear that's a good sign and when the drainage is below 50 ml that's also good), and I went for a shower and got dressed. Kirsteen also enabled me to remove the plaster cos I asked (don't tell my surgeon, it had been stuck on by a sealing gun I think!) and to see the scar (as my surgeon promised, the scar's a smiley face!) and then she replaced the plaster. Then we chose a softee and stuck it in my bra. My bras are still underwired and the wire is sore on the scar, I have tried the

---

[14] Softees are a small foam breast form covered in cotton material to put in your bra as a temporary measure. It was only later that someone suggested I could have pinned it in place using a safety pin!

softee in my support vests, purchased by my personal shopper Kristin, but to be honest I'm happy without at the moment and am considering going without. This will possibly cure a lot of guys from staring at my chest, if not any woman's chest, and hopefully cured them of staring at my chest as well.

I talked to my Mum about this last night. I have always been able to talk to my Mum. We don't always see eye to eye, but I can always talk to her. For me it will also give me more fun in calibrating people's reactions – I notice some people don't visit me, as they don't know what to say (I've been here before, after Michael died some people avoided me for a year or more, as they 'didn't know what to say'). What to say is 'how are you?' (leave out the 'feeling' word), then listen to the answer and take it from there. Any useful advice you might have is not useful, unless of course you have had a mastectomy. I mean things like 'you should be resting', 'he should be doing it all for you' (he does the housework, but I'm not totally incapacitated and I'm presenting in 11 days time!) 'Should you be out?' (I'll come back to 'should' later.) Ah yes, and the wrong opening file phrase 'In this difficult time for you' – that is from my GP surgery, the NHS likes to keep you ill. Wait until I'm typing with two hands!

I did have a few tears on my own in the shower room, but they really were tears of joy, that I'm alive!

116

Anyway Sunday 1st March I got out of hospital, the sun was shining and all's right with the world.

11th March 2009: This convalescing lark

What now?

Well I've written to *Loose Women* and as you will know I asked you all to write to them too, no response from them, yet! I also appear to be writing articles for other people's websites – I think this is good.

But let's go back to being at home.

Gee, it was great to be back home, even though lying flat on my back is not necessarily my fave sleeping position, no one wakes me up to take my blood pressure – why do they do this, do people realise torture does exist in this country, meted out by nurses? However, getting up and sitting in front of the PC is good for my back, it stretches it out! Jim made butternut squash soup last Monday, excellent especially when you consider this is a beef farmer! We went for a short walk, by the time we got out: (a) it was late, (b) we got ambushed by the neighbours who told me I 'should be resting', and then (c) it blew a gale, but at least I'd been out. My walks have become progressively longer and I can now make it up to the High Street (going up hill was a problem, my chest was saying no, no we're not joined up yet) – I can in fact make it all by myself and I went shopping by myself today. I have been deserted all day for the second time this week and Jim's mobile phone is who knows where cos he hasn't rung me! (Correction he has just phoned – just before 'knocking off' for the day). I also managed to get out when the neighbours were napping; no one rescued me and brought me back!

Tuesday morning last week, Kristin arrived with some support vests, and spent some time with me, grown up without small boys. She also tinted my eyebrows; I had wondered where they were going!

I thought I'd died or my chest had split last Tuesday evening when I made some daft attempt in my sleep to turn over in a way I couldn't – I lay there for a while, then gingerly touched my left side, it felt dry, a while later I gingerly got up and went out into the hall to check my dressing was still white, it was – yippee! I honestly thought I fallen apart.

There is this thing, as I know some people have missed it, cos I can email etc. I have had major surgery, someone cut through muscles, sinews, nerves etc. and they are jangling their way back together and it's going to take a while which is why I have a sick note for at least 6 weeks and I can feel every single little hole in the road on the passenger side in the car – err, not nice.

Wednesday we managed a longer walk even though I was nursing a sore chest, not that these walks are far. My breast care nurse phoned to ask how I was. Hasn't phoned since.

Thursday was the day we had Leon who was reportedly ill! He came with his own lunch which he shared with Jim and shared my lunch by taking it home as his lunch for the following day, and he moaned (about the things I said no to and the things he couldn't have).

Sleeping is improving, and rubbing St John's Wort oil on the jangly bits under my armpit helps.

Friday we shopped in Findhorn and Lidl – hey these are highlights,

I've discovered *Hill Street Blues* is on daytime TV too – this will mean little to the younger ones of you reading this ☺

Saturday I decided we needed to go to Elgin, one of my shoes was there – in the shoe repairers before you think any other thoughts. We went briefly onto the High Street and then to TKMaxx, where I tried on three tops, mmm a bit flat looking, and over-the-head tops are taxing to put on, I can tell you! So we went to the new New Look store. Jim took one look at the store, went into panic and remained at the bottom of the stairs propping up the staircase, which was fortunate. I went upstairs, had Jim ventured up there, there are seats. However I chose a short-sleeved buttoned-down-the-front top to try on (on the principle button down the front is easier to get on and off than over the head (less stretching upwards – very important) and a

120

big check shirt with press studs on the front. Fortunately as I was looking around, my 'personal shopper' arrived, Kristin works there part time, she had arrived at work and encountered Jim propping up the staircase and gone upstairs to find me. I had just brought what I thought was the next size shirt into the changing room and it transpired it was actually a size smaller (no wonder they were reduced – dodgy sizing) and I couldn't get it off my arms as I didn't have the flexibility – 'err Kristin help,' and she did, rescuing me and getting me another shirt. I wasn't quite ready to face a strange person in a changing room and try to explain why I couldn't get out of the shirt and them to notice I only had one boob (this has since changed).

Sunday started out beautiful weather, then it snowed – up here we have four seasons, no not a pizza, no not by Verdi, four seasons in one day, we certainly had them all on Sunday. However, we then went for a walk to Findhorn Bay (we drove there first), it was a brief walk, as the tide was in and being near to full moon it's extreme weather time of the month and there was a very blustery gale – we went to the Bakehouse Café, mm delicious soya cappuccino made with some obscure coffee substitute for me (!) and for Jim the real thing cappuccino and a scone (had he looked in the glass case, he probably would have had the world's gooey-est cake – but he'll do that next time – novice). I saw someone I know through business, gosh he's married with a daughter, was a long time since I'd seen him last. Then we went to Lidl (exciting life I lead – but you never know what you might find in there! – biker jackets next week – hmmm, I just might). The rest of the day was pretty tame, as no one phoned or visited – sigh and Jim disappeared into the conservatory, no prizes for guessing what he was doing in there on a Sunday!

Monday this week I was deserted and grumpy, I slept badly the previous night. I did some tidying and a little dusting (must have been bored, when do I do housework? I have a man for that). I had wanted to attempt to get to the post box with a letter, was just about to go when Jim came home, so we went together, he tripped near the duck pond, not me!

Tuesday was more exciting – Kristin came on the train as her car was playing up, so still under warranty she took it to the garage, was good to talk. Just as she was trying the Easter wreath on for size (on her head – and she wonders why Nico recently put his nappy on his head!) Malcolm arrived to pick up the key for the Practice Group I normally run – Kristin commented 'the wreath is egg–cellent!' Malcolm, one of my Associates, was overcome at how well I looked, me sporting new shirt from New Look and Wonderwoman T-shirt – reminded him 'strong stuff this NLP' and thanked him for compliment. Rebecca then arrived en route back from Aberdeen.

Anyway Jim took Kristin back to Elgin and they purchased a PowerPoint for Dummies book for me (which solved my PowerPoint issues in 20 seconds, what a saving) and Rebecca and I went to Findhorn (as in the Park) for lunch and to shop ☺ Prior to that I had a telephone interview with the *Press & Journal* – 'Now, will they print that?' I ask myself. (They didn't).

Today I've written an article for *Mum and Me* about 'My Left Breast' and the boob photo will be revealed to the public (not quite and not published until October 2010).

Oh yes, and for those of you who have read the book *Finding The Relationship You Deserve*: page 10, point 25 started our day – might be too much information for some, but for some people reading this now or in the future it might be something they just want to know. Nothing hurt, nothing dropped off and it was fun ☺

My compelling purpose

So I explained earlier how I built my compelling purpose and on 19th March I went to the hairdressers, had the grey covered over and then we went to Aberdeen. I put on my new brown trousers, my new top and the red jacket. We were in plenty of time as Jim starts to worry in places he doesn't know and also any town larger than Inverness really! We arrived nice and early and, well, over-welcomed (it was great that everyone was so pleased to see me). I was photographed (later Kristin remarked I looked as if I had shrunk, I pointed out well no boob to fill the clothes, our clothes are made to fit round a shape which includes boobs), kissed and looked after. I'd eaten before I left, ah yes I haven't mentioned that I've changed my eating habits.

The presentation went extremely well, the applause was thunderous, and hopefully we have some more people interested in NLP.

One thing I was asked was to read out the statement for Breast Cancer Care, that was not part of my original remit and I found that hard, as I had to read it (because I didn't know it) and that meant looking down. Looking down tears will flow more easily, so I had to keep looking up to blink back the tears.

Try it – when you 'feel sad' look up and see something you like or look for 'that special shade of blue' in the sky.

Exercising or regaining movement!

As I mentioned previously, the only contact I had with a physiotherapist was when one appeared on the ward on the Friday very briefly as she was in a hurry (she said she had been to see me the day before, but I wasn't there!) and gave me leaflet with exercises and told me it was too soon for me to start and she would be back on Monday (she'll have been disappointed then!).

Well I did the exercises on my own at home (no follow-up here). I understand from my friend Margit (and others) in Germany that there women go into a convalescent home after a mastectomy or lumpectomy and are given physio, and taken through breathing and movement exercises for a period of 4 weeks! As well as any other treatment they may be having.

One of the exercises, walking your fingers up the wall and moving closer is particularly painful, I'm curious if a lot of women give up on this one. I went to see my Pilates teacher Sara Hunt, in her studio for a private session. This took place 1 day short of 3 weeks after my operation. I'd bought a book from Amazon, *The Breast Cancer Survivor's' Fitness Plan*: in that it says start exercising after 4 weeks. Well, I was wanting to do more and, above all, do something for my back as sleeping on the same side all the time was hard on my back. What had stopped me was the question 'If I get down on the floor, how do I get up again?' So I went to see Sara, I showed her the leaflet and the book and I showed her my scar, hey what she doesn't know about bodies isn't worth knowing and from her I learned that Pilates and your Pilates teacher are there to be adapted (in the correct manner) for your body and she makes it all delicious ('delicious' in Sara's 'model of the world' is not the same as mine, but it's a great word for the sensation that might otherwise be 'it hurts'). So together with me, Sara worked out a routine that stretched my back out, increased my range of arm movement – and I could get up and down off the floor, after a little help from her it was easy actually. And I did this every morning from then on, I think my class thinks I'm either joking or a creep, but I want 'to live for ever'.

It certainly made a huge difference to my mobility. The interested glances I got when I went back to breast care centre to have fluid removed showed that!

Oh yes, just before I went for my first post-op appointment, Friday 13th March (did I also mention the day on which I first saw my surgeon, 30th January, was the feast day of the patron saint St Aldegundis who actually died as a result of breast cancer in 684 at the age of 45 – not to be confused with Saint Agatha whose feast day is 5th February, she had her breasts cut off by the Romans).[15] So yes – post-op appointment – I still had on the dressing (the one the nurse put on for me in the hospital before I left, because I asked to see the scar, and the dressing was itchy and coming off) and I had looked down at the dressing area and in passing wondered if my boob was growing back. It turned out it was fluid, now no one was forthcoming about this fluid, apart from the area being also a bit hot and itchy (more on that later). I assume it might have been lymph fluid but no one actually told me that. The fluid was drained away and I was told if it comes back in, just phone and come in and we'll drain it off.

The fluid came back and I duly went back again, a third time when the whole thing was hot and itchy and slightly raised at one side, I went back again. This time I saw the other breast care nurse. She examined me and said 'oh it's healing' and I said 'okay'. She looked at me amazed, apart from having looked on whilst I got undressed unaided (I can do that, I practised getting my left arm above my head even in the hospital). 'Ah well,' I said 'my Mum was a nurse, she often said if something was hot and itchy it was healing so that's okay.' And it was, and as soon as I knew it was just healing, the whole area started to calm down.

---

[15] And if you are collecting more trivia, Wendy Richard (Pauline Fowler in *Eastenders*) died on the day I had my mastectomy. End of trivia here.

128

I also rubbed to begin with golden calendula oil into the scar and later wild rose oil and certainly at the time of writing it's nice and flat and smooth. I have a 'fatty' bit under my arm, my breast care nurse explained normally my breast would keep that more taut, so I want to work on flattening that bit.

Now swimming. I was itching to get back to swimming; one thing that stopped me was not driving (swimming pools not very accessible unless you have transport where I live). Then before I went back to work we went on holiday to the Red Sea, now there's a story. I chose a resort with a swimming pool and also its own beach as I wanted to get in some swimming in the warm. Again, like getting down on the floor, I was worried about getting in the pool. Now before Christmas 2008 I had been having lessons to learn the crawl (no one ever taught me), so I phoned my swimming teacher Ian Parfitt.[16] We had two sessions before I went away, Ian got me swimming on my back and then gentle breast stroking and then he said 'you know Rosie, you could go snorkelling', so we tried that out in the pool and some exercise as well. And when I got to Sharm el Sheikh I did buy a mask, snorkel tube and flippers and I went snorkelling. Thank you Ian, it was mind blowing – hey so I had had cancer I had no idea that would lead to swimming in my own aquarium. I also bought a cheap disposable underwater

---

[16] www.mandianswimmingschool.co.uk: if nothing else, visit his website to see the bubbles that appear!

camera, Nico and I looked through twenty-seven photos of fish and he said twenty-seven times 'No, Nemo not there.' I'll be able to take him to look for Nemo himself one day!

Back home I started riding my bike, last year's birthday present and I've hardly been out on it, so building up stamina is interesting and I'm a fair weather or light wind rider. Pilates: I went back to my class with the others, annoyed at times my arm won't go where I want it to, Sara reminds me I have had a major op!

23rd April 2009: This prosthesis thing, breast form, chicken fillet!

Well I got my false boob last week. The Breast Care nurses said I needed to bring a bra for the boob fitting; the bra shop said I needed to bring the boob to get a bra – ah, clarity again. I needed to buy a bra, as I had previously had underwired bras (there is some school of thought that says these cause breast cancer!). So I purchased a bra, non-wired, and got my boob on Thursday 16th April, I then wore boob all day and into the evening as I went Eden Court Theatre in Inverness with my friend David T to watch Buddy. I clapped and clapped and clapped, making my muscles quite sore and the next day when I wore the boob again my 'breast' area was a little sore, so I put it back in its cradle (it comes in a plastic insert in which it sits when not in use, inside a cardboard box, all very tasteful). I bought another bra as the first one holds boob in place well and seems ok apart from some odd 'itching' sensations which I have yet to discover if that's still the healing or the boob next the skin. The second bra, whilst being more comfortable as a bra, allows boob to slip, not a lot and I'm sure no one notices, most people don't even notice there is no boob there.

Pocketed bras it seems cannot be purchased in shops, well I haven't found one up here yet, and I can order them from a shop. Now, you might be saying 'order online', well so far I have tried that, all the ones I like or want are either out of stock or not in my size! And in the case of one manufacturer who claims they 'provide a range of products and services that have helped thousands of women to concentrate on getting back to normal' so that you don't feel completely alone, their customer service is non-existent online. So I have ordered two pockets to sew in from a completely different manufacturer[17] after Googling – the lady in the bra shop does not know you can just order pockets – and I've ordered a bra from eBay. We are off on holiday to Egypt and I suspect my boob will be too hot to wear there, so although it's travelling with us, I'll only wear it at night I think. I don't feel alone, I feel frustrated and I'm sure that's not just because I live in what shipping companies regard as a remote area (only remote cos they don't have the remotest idea where we are). It just brings me back to previous thoughts on perhaps not wearing the thing. We shall see.

I showed Leon and Nico the boob on the Saturday, Nico 2 days away from being 3 years old seemingly required three or four looks at boob and Granny's 'ow'. After his last look he walked off and said (he has just started to talk sentences, big brother gets in the way), 'Granny 'at booby, no yum yum.' The powers of deduction at nearly 3!

---

[17] www.conturabelle.co.uk.

The boob is cold to touch at first, but quickly feels the right temperature both against the skin and to touch, until I take it out of the bra and then it cools down again, it's quite a pleasant thing and feels ok and I don't notice when it's there, apart from suddenly there is something where for 7 weeks there was a space. Also this one is the same size as my real right boob; my late left boob was always slightly smaller, I could have had a slightly smaller one, but after advice from my breast care nurse (more later) I opted for a same-size one. I dislike the word 'prosthesis', partly I suppose as it could be any kind of prosthesis!

The 16th April was also a great day, as on the way back form the hospital and obtaining the 'breast form' we stopped at a local farm and I saw my first lamb being born. Amazing how that little thing is compelled to get up and start moving on its wobbly legs and it takes us humans so long!

Thoughts and experiences with breast forms

I agreed to having a first breast form that was the same size as my remaining boob. That was a mistake; it got in the way, funny how that slight size difference made a difference. After about 5 months I went back and had a smaller one fitted. It was also a different shape, more of a triangle which is my boob shape.

I found even though most mastectomy bras have a cotton pocket (some of the cheaper ones have nylon) that I got a bit sweaty when out either in the sun or sometimes when out in large gatherings of people. I then found Amoena[18] produce a bra with a cotton wicking-covered insert with cooling gel inside, so that you can place it in the fridge. The North of Scotland hasn't been so hot of late that I've needed to do that, but the new boob has made a whole heap of difference in many ways: (a) it's cooler and I don't feel sticky and (b) I discovered that M&S make post-surgery bras, no pocket but a better fit, so the Amoena Climate, as this breast form is called, slips in the bra, fits snug to my chest and when I look down (I've spoken to other women about this – we think others can tell we have a breast form in a pocket – others can't and don't see the pocket – ok I can't wear low-cut tops, but then I never wanted to and still don't, other people see your boobs and low-cut top rather

---

[18] www.amoena.com.

134

than you first) I only see the snug-fitting bra. Not only that, the M&S bra is comfy and cheaper than others. Well done M&S!

The Red Sea

Had you told me on 26th December 2008 (when I was on way back from Market Harborough, in Leicester) that 2009 was to be, what is so far the case, the most exciting year of my life, so far, I would have asked, 'How?' Well, I had plans. We saw in the New Year in Benidorm, Jim and I and some other well-behaved people at a quiet hotel. We had two New Years, one Spanish time and one UK time (we would have been fine with once). On 5th January we saw the Three Kings arrive in Benidorm and hundreds upon hundreds of people forming a procession to mark this important event in Spain. Spanish children receive one present on 6th January (Epiphany, when the Wise Man arrived in Bethlehem to visit the infant Jesus) and this is their Christmas present, perhaps they understand more about the meaning of Christmas than some children and some of their families in the UK? (I digress).

We returned home on 6th January and on the 7th I received my letter heralding the unexpected changes to my 2009, my Plans, my Goals, my Resolutions.

So here we are, Compelling Purposes set no. 3 (no. 1 was discarded, no. 2 carried out).

I sat writing this on a beach in Sharm el Sheikh. Yes, this is a hot country (I've never really done heat before). It is, in case you don't know, in Asia on the Sinai peninsular, in the Asian part of Egypt. I really liked it here and the Egyptians here in the resort were so polite and helpful.

On 26th April I went snorkelling. I was just a few feet from the fish and swimming in an aquarium. It was fantastic. I've also been swimming twice in the pool and snorkelling again this morning. I've had two hot-stone Bedouin massages and a facial using 'threading' – amazing.

Next day, the Pyramids at Giza. All this and 60 days ago I had my breast removed. You know life gives us amazing opportunities – if we want to take them.

The swimming is about preventing problems, stretching and mobilising the muscles – it's also starting Goal no. 2 that's about getting thinner. And here, where we are staying, there's plenty of opportunity to walk around the complex!

The Pyramids were amazing. We left the hotel at 4.30 a.m. and finally flew from Cairo airport at 8 a.m. Early morning Cairo is incredible in the rush hour, so many people, so many cars, old cars, traffic rules non-existent, people everywhere and it's incredibly dirty (well it hardly ever rains). After a hair-raising drive, we see in the distance the Pyramids! And lots of haze (it turned out that was pollution, it burns off around 2 p.m.!). The Pyramids are just truly awesome, we had a hilarious camel ride to the Middle Pyramid, hilarious cos I was petrified at the thought of getting off the camel as it went up in the air – quite frankly it's a long way up there! Also camels appear not to look where they are going.

After some wondering and wandering around between the Middle Pyramid and Great Pyramid we were then bussed to the Sphinx. Amazing! and we were so lucky our guide took some great photos. Later we went to the Museum of Antiquities and saw the Tutankhamen exhibition – again speechless.

I had no idea that I would even want to go to Egypt and I guess what I will go again. There's good and bad in everything.

Oh hell – other people – it's me who had the cancer!

In the last month, I have been a little confused by comments such as 'I can't believe how well you look!' I am supposed to look how? Does no one believe me I'm fine!

'How are you psychologically?' I didn't know what that meant until I asked a business client of mine, with whom I get on well. Psychologically? What does that mean? And he said quite simply, 'well when my ex-wife had a hysterectomy, she had problems coming to terms with loss of part of femininity.' Ah, no. I have already talked about this to a few people, they usually ask me 'how's your partner about this?' Well firstly they are my boobs and secondly I tell people he's actually a bum man, retired farmer spent a lot of time patting cow's backsides, well that's what I tell myself when he pats mine and I smile, he's showing me he cares (took me a while to get used to this way of behaving).[19]

My friend Sam Welsh and I have recorded a chat for The Strong Breast Revolution at the Edinburgh festival and we talk about our boobs and our relationship with them and how it's us who are important.

---

[19] See *Finding the Relationship You Deserve* in respect of other people sometimes doing or liking things we don't and that could be okay, as long as it doesn't hurt us in any way.

Sam asked me on this recording, 'do you miss the boob?' 'Well,' I answered, 'you know the only time I've been missing it is when I get dry after coming out of the bath or the shower, then as I pull the towel up to dry under my left boob, oops, the towel slips upwards on the left and I realise there's no boob there!' We also talked about the bingo dress. Do you know what a bingo dress is? I once lived in Middlesbrough (you either like Middlesbrough or you don't – let's not go there) and I bought what was probably my first-ever low-cleavage dress, in about (well no, exactly) 1985; it was black with white spots, very stylish for the era ☺ Bingo dress? Yes, you know eyes down and look in! Well I can't wear one of those any more, because the mastectomy bras are designed to cover the breast form and therefore, sight of breast form or bra would be interesting, to say the least, in the bingo dress ☺ I was never really that comfortable with showing my boobs (well apart from in private), I'm not so bothered now, but there at times when I'm networking, training or even sitting on a bus, when I'd like (a) people to concentrate on the message and (b) to have control of who looks down my frock, so no bingo dress. And I'm sort of that age, girls, when showing your bra straps as so many ladies do nowadays was frowned upon. My granny, bless her cotton gloves and cigarette holder, would have a fit (several fits actually) – 'cover yourself up girl'. That's just me. Having said that I'd be quite happy for people to see photos of me or even be on stage in a 'controlled' atmosphere so that people can see what a mastectomy looks like and also my very nice, smiley face scar. Sam thinks I might have fangs tattooed on it, I think just some eyes and a nose – don't tempt me ☺ Someone else did mention the world had to be careful that I didn't 'whip the breast form out in Tesco and run down the aisles with it' (unlikely as I am anti-Tesco).[20]

I have discovered there was a rumour in Aberdeen that I was very ill, and in Highlands and Islands I haven't been seen around, so either I'd gone out of business or I was ill and gone out of business.

---

[20] Ah well, just after I got the Amoena Climate, I went into Tesco to get a Costa Coffee and bumped into Chris who had been on the ward with me and showed her the new breast form: we both peeked down my top ☺

Employment Support Allowance

Now this is the new name for the state benefit you will get if you have paid sufficient contributions and you can't work. Be warned the powers that be go out of their way to put you in the belief that you will not get anything!

First you need to speak to someone on the phone. The initial person I spoke to was very frosty and this, a couple of days after coming out of hospital, was not very pleasant. There then followed a phone interview for around 30 or 40 minutes; this guy was very pleasant and said I could stop at any time. But the language on the information sheet from the Job Centre is if you don't claim within so many days then you might not get anything or you might lose out.

Then there's this double-edged sword for the self-employed. There's something called a 'Pathways back to work' interview which comes after you have been off for a certain amount of time. Now this comes irrespective of the fact that you have a mastectomy, in fact I've discovered lots of people don't know what this mastectomy is – 'I've had me boob off!' Now the medical profession seems to think you should be off for 8 weeks or more, and I can understand why, as it was a large lump of flesh and several bits of muscle etc. and if I concentrate on the submodalities of pain and not those of getting better, I could stay off longer. Now if you were employed before, you are permitted to work 16 hours without this affecting your state benefit. If you are self-employed you are allowed to earn zilch, zero, nada. I can only conjecture that is because the self-employed earn shed loads of money and would therefore not need help from the state! So I had myself 'signed off' (or something like that) – I was able to do this over the phone (my psychological state was questioned, not that I understood that at the time, I said 'that's fine'). And there I was, no safety net. And then I discovered that various things had not happened as I had perhaps assumed (never assume anything – I spend a lot of time saying that), because I had been concentrating on getting well. Silly me. Ho hum.

Fortunately we don't have a mortgage or dependent children so getting back on my self-employed feet does not mean those things won't be paid for. I recently heard from a colleague of someone who has a mortgage and he is watching his business disappear so that his mortgage is paid because he can't receive any benefits if he starts working again!!!

Am I wrong in thinking something is wrong here?

Now you cannot argue with the government; in fact, I was sent a final demand for 10 (ten) pence (yes) that had been underpaid into my National Insurance in error by the government. Just for the hell of it (it was a free phone number) I phoned and asked for it to be written off, collected in some other way. I asked 'isn't it a little ridiculous to chase this (and it's a government error) amount of money?' After all, the postage alone for the letter I received was more than 10 pence. Any commercial organisation would have as part of their computer program some way of writing this kind of amount off and not sending the letter out (I would hope – it makes economic sense). So I phoned and was met with a firm and incredulous answer that I would have to pay otherwise any future benefits might be affected. Friends suggested I send in 10 one-pence pieces, but that wasn't allowed, it must be paid at a bank or by bank transfer. In fact, the lady on the other end of the phone thought it was quite ok to take the 10 pence into a bank. I capitulated and paid my 10 pence – by bank transfer.

'When my granny had two boobs!'

Leon now has a new reference point; it began when Kristin drove the boys to Aberdeen to spend the weekend with me at the flat. Seemingly he said 'you know we went here, when my Granny had two boobs'. A lot of things are prefaced by 'when you had two boobs'.

We recently went to a local school May Fair, as we drove up the approach road, a voice came from the back of the car 'I's been here before, when my Granny had two boobs!' A second voice followed (this is Shannon, also 5), 'You know my Granny has lost a boob.' Yes indeed, she had last year. Now interestingly, I haven't 'lost' the boob. I know fine and well where it went it and I gave it up willingly, in the knowledge and belief that doing so was a good thing to do, for me. If you try those words out, does it make a difference?

NLP is sometimes dubbed as 'Positive Thinking'. Personally I think 'Positive Thinking' is a bit of a catch phrase and you can always assume that someone is doing something for Positive Reasons and that they are a Positive Person. I would like to admit here, I gave up that boob because I wanted to avoid radiotherapy. How can someone blasting me with gamma rays be doing something that is healthy to me or for me? And since I took that decision I have heard of many side effects of what happens. You know, dear healthcare peeps, just because we've

145

doing it this way for years why is good for me? I really would not have been persuaded to have either radiotherapy or chemotherapy because it 'might' help. I really do like my changes to what I eat, so no red meat: I don't miss it and I have tried it. No cow's cheese: well, I often had some odd reaction to cheese, I do occasionally eat goat's cheese or buffalo mozzarella or some veggie type cheese (not convinced by that). Sugar or artificial substitutes aren't good for anyone, how could they be? They taste nice for one thing.

How do I do this, change my thoughts about things that are not good for me? Well I turn down the sub-modalities. (What? more soon.) I also know as well that some people have success with EFT (Emotional Freedom Technique). This works best if you are a very touchy, feely person. Preferably find a properly trained practitioner of EFT, who is also a properly trained practitioner of NLP[21] and work on your cravings to use NLP with food (more on this later).

Before that, a little on motivation . . .

---

[21] www.professionalguildofnlp.com for NLP or www.anlp.org for ANLP (The Association for NLP) professionals. The Professional Guild requires your practitioner or even better well-trained master practitioner to have 120 hours of training as a practitioner.

NLP stuff: It's fine to be a 'Positive Person' or a 'Negative Nelly'

NLP talks about Meta Programmes and Shelle Rose Charvet, in her book *Words That Change Minds*, uses the Language and Behaviour Profile, which was based on the Meta Programmes originally. These patterns are the higher level filters we use (in NLP, anything that is a higher level, out of consciousness, is known as 'Meta'), and these filters drive us to do something, or not. For me the beauty of the Meta Programmes is that the two ends of each extreme of a Meta Programme are places we might be at, at different times in our lives, of the year, even of the day. Recently I received a phone call from a colleague who said 'he was feeling a little self-indulgent today'. (Now there is a little information missing there, because to me self-indulgent is eating chocolate or some such and I had to check what he meant). He meant he 'was wallowing in self-pity', his words. He, like me, is mostly a very positive person.

For some of us, I know very positive people can be very annoying, and so can people who act in the opposite manner be for us very positive people – and it's fine to be who we are. That's a great fact we can learn from NLP, it's fine to be a 'Positive Person' or a 'Negative Nelly' because there is a great deal to be gained and learned from both places. What is also great is to realise that we can change the way we react, if we

147

want to or need to. Also sometimes it's more useful to change the way I am behaving in a particular situation, and other times it would be useful to change my language so that I can enable those people who are not 'working with me' or 'who are working against me' to work with me.

So, a question: are you clear about what you want, and are you motivated and energised by 'what you will achieve', '. . . have', '. . . accomplish' or '. . . get'? Do you want to know about the 'advantages', the 'benefits'? Or do you always, or just, or more often than not, see or hear or feel things about what you don't want and 'want to avoid', '. . . prevent', '. . . eliminate', do you 'notice the problems first'? Or is it that there are people around you who fall into one of those categories and those people really annoy you?

Well both types of people are okay; different people just think about things in different ways, they filter differently. In a team it's important to have a balance of people (and this includes your team at home). If you only ever have people who work towards achievements, the things they will get, the advantages, etc., it could be that they will forget to risk plan, forget to have a contingency plan, to have enough reserves in the bank to pay the bills, etc. If you only ever have people who notice problems, you may never get started. So a balance is needed, as well as a dialogue and an understanding that Fred is motivated in this manner and Doreen in this manner. Otherwise Fred may start to worry if Doreen consistently 'finds fault'.

Currently, on a course I have been running for 7 months, all the participants are both Moving Towards and Moving Away From, so they are noticing their achievements and what they have accomplished (Towards), as well as noticing what they have avoided, got rid of (Away From). All, that is, bar one – when I get feedback forms at the end of the weekend, all bar one rate the whole weekend at 100–110%. The one hovers around 80% and covers every available bit of the A4 sheet and sometimes the other page with the problems – these problems are so trivial at times – the chairs, the coffee, or ones over which we have no control 'so and so didn't turn up' (they were ill, it snowed and the trains didn't run) – that you might start to wonder 'is this person who concentrates on those things on a different course?' However, their life has a strong 'Moving Away From' pattern, their life consists of problems, things they must solve, avoid, eliminate, go out of his way to get away from (according to them). In their job, which is working for a major oil company, this will stand them in good stead. In everyday life with other people however, possibly not, which is why it is sometimes useful to appreciate how I think and the words that I use, perhaps I might change the way I act at home to save my personal relationship.

On the other hand, we have all met people at times who only ever see everything as being good, there are a great many newly converted or 'born again' NLPers who are often a little like that, some of them helped delay my first foray into NLP as I didn't want to tell everyone how wonderful it is and what you will achieve (and I am Moving Towards in the main!), because I recognised, and didn't know why at the time, that some people are put off by this, what seems to them to be over-positive stuff.

We all meet people like this – how can we work with them, either as friends and family or at work and in the medical world? (and where are they mostly coming from?)

Well, let's start with: How can you check where they are operating from?

1. Had you asked me 'What is important to you about your breast cancer treatment?', I would have said 'living, no side effects and being well'.

2. You could then have asked me 'And what's important to you about living?', and I would have said 'I have a hell of a lot to do, places to go, people to meet, things I promised myself I would do and I have two grandsons who I want to be there for as a positive memory.'

3. Or you could have asked me 'And what's important to you about "no side effects"?', and I would have said 'Well mostly the same as above, but (aha) essentially I am a coward and I hate pain [think about this in light of some of the things you have previously read in this book]! I want a quality of life over which I have control and if it goes belly up I'm happy to take the blame (yes really). I've also seen some of the side effects of medication in my family and experienced some on me too (partly why I was overweight). And I'm a busy woman. And I want to be well.'

So my first answer tells you 'I want to live', which is possibly Moving Towards, and it also tells you I'm Moving Away From 'side effects' and being unwell (the opposite of 'being well'). So I'm a bit of both, a Positive Person and a Negative Nelly.

The first answer doesn't always tell you whether someone is moving away from (so avoiding) or towards (thinking about what they gain, achieve) in a particular context, so either take the single answer they give you or, if they give you a list, take one.

What is important here is you now need to ask a further question or questions because in this age of permanent and pervasive Positive Thinking, the first answer from Moving Away people will possibly be positive (as we come to believe we have to say something positive, even if things are not). It's what happens next that gives you the pattern – ask them 'Why is that important?', and continue if necessary. One example comes from people often talking about freedom (in fact when Jo Pirie and I run Money Coaching courses with NLP, Jo has Financial Freedom as one thing that many people want and talk about): you need to check whether this is freedom from 'debt', 'living in rented accommodation', 'working in the job I have' or freedom to 'go on holiday', 'write a book', 'spend time with friends and family' etc.

Certain businesses, organisations and families run towards or away from models (where do you think the medical model is?): it might be appropriate for them. Do they prevent something from happening? Does the person you are speaking to only want to know about what he/she will avoid? If so, then tell them about that and not about the advantages. Check it out, sometimes people present advantages to me in the form of moving away from (so what I will avoid), that does not work for me on its own – I need then to know about the advantages.

There's also a good little technique you can use for yourself or with someone else. If you often find yourself Moving Towards something or Moving Away From something and you want to know why or you might want or have to change that. Imagine a line, or draw one on a sheet of A4 or A3, or imagine one on the floor which you can walk along (perhaps in the privacy of your own home or office) and think about this client, project, issue, problem, opportunity or achievement that you have been moving towards or away from. At one end of the line is Moving Away From, at the other end is Moving Towards, physically or mentally stand on, or place your finger, or coin, or small piece of paper on this line at the place where you think you might be now in respect of this client, project, issue, problem, opportunity or achievement you have been moving towards or away from. Then moving yourself, or the counter, or piece of paper towards or away from the other end of the line, notice what you see, hear and feel at each stage as you move along the line and how the client, project, issue, problem, opportunity or achievement changes and what new information you gather and how you might do things differently or walk away and leave things as they are.

NLP stuff: Submodalities

Think of submodalities as tiny changes in the representational systems as we process internally (or occasionally externally, as in 'seeing red'). So what you see may be big, small, close, far away, dull, bright, moving, still, etc. What you hear may be loud, soft, shrill, soothing, behind you, inside or outside, etc. What you feel may be still, moving, warm, cool, pointed, dull, outside, inside, etc. These differences seem to be the means by which we keep our external behaviour reasonably consistent.

Think about two of your friends, one of whom is your best friend, and the other of whom is your nearly best friend. How do you know, without thinking about it or consciously adjusting yourself, how to greet each of them, to reflect your slightly different feelings for them? Submodalities seem to be the answer. We appear to have a 'filing system' where we keep almost all of our internal information, and it is coded by submodalities to tell us where to find it, and how to respond to it. We file things such as people, beliefs, reality, school subjects we 'can do', and things we 'have to do'. These systems are individual and unique. Indeed sometimes, one person's system is opposite to another's. One person may keep people they don't trust large, close up, colours bright, and noisy. Another person may keep people they don't trust small, far away, dull and quiet. What seems to be the case, though, is that we are each consistent in our own filing system.

There are a number of other implications of a system of submodalities. Someone who has the same internal coding for things that really happen and things they imagine have happened, will have little sense of reality. People who have the same coding for 'have to do' as they do for something they 'could do' are unlikely to be dependable in their promises. So sometimes the absence of a desired behaviour may be due to the absence of the necessary coding or file!

Sometimes we simply mis-file people or information, perhaps because of the way in which we originally received and perceived the message. This is why it is so harmful to most people when a teacher says, 'Lots of you may find this difficult.' Whatever comes next is filed by many people as 'difficult' and as a result, they find it more difficult to do it! And we could use this system well by eliciting the appropriate submodalities for an experience, and slipping in our communication, knowing that it will be appropriately filed!

(For this so far, my thanks go to a lady called Cricket Kemp, who gave me that as part of my NLP Practitioner manual.)

Now, you can change the submodalities of food. After all, if people are appealing and not good for us, what stops us from making food less appealing? If you've ever given anything up, you will have already used this kind of technique in some way, so you could work that out. What did you change around chocolate, wine, cigarettes? Can you work that out?

Some tips and hints on smoking: if it's the taste that's so inviting, then what is it about the taste? Is there a point at which you no longer like the taste? Do you like the smell on your clothes, your hands? Your breath? Do you like the taste in your mouth next morning? Do you like the coughing? Do you like the feeling of tightness in your chest when you walk fast or run?

What is it about smoking that you like? And what is it about smoking you dislike?

So if you like the smell of the tobacco and you hate the taste in your mouth later, then every time you smell the tobacco, fast forward your sense to the taste in your mouth, the prickling on your tongue, the 'old ashtray' taste and turn that up. Practise, practise, and practise a little more and you will then succeed in resisting the urge, be warned it takes at least 30 days for nicotine to leave your system so you have to hang on in there.

Chocolate or cakes? Next time you see a bar of chocolate or a cake in shop, think of this – imagine the chocolate (or cake) the luscious irresistible taste, as you open your mouth and take the first bite. Imagine biting into it and taking it into your mouth, then after you have chewed it well, swallow and notice how it slides down your gullet and into your stomach. Once in your stomach, it's met by all the digestive acids and the other contents of your stomach, it turns into a brown mass covered in acids and goo. See it down there, hear it gurgling, notice what it might taste like now. Would you want it now? As it turns into poor-quality sugars and fats?

You can do similar things with other foods and addictions. You can notice how bright and inviting some things appear to your mind (and stomach) and turn the submodalities down, make them dark, dull, uninviting. For things that you perhaps might be better off eating, turn the submodalities up a little; think about what the long-term effect of eating healthily will be for you. Act 'as if' you are healthy. What's that like? What do you do? What can you do better? What can you see yourself doing? What do others see you doing? What will others say about you? What will you say about you? How will you feel?

Time to decide

The following is written as the way I see, think about and feel about things (as is the majority of this book) – in particular in respect of my self-employment.

This wondrous thing called hindsight: I think that the 30 days between my diagnosis and the op was far too short a time, given the weeks of recovery which follow, the need to know more about treatment available, and the definite need to have a proper, executable plan for the patient's life post op. (Trust me, this is about the patient – so many relatives think it's about the relative.)

I honestly don't know if other women are given any help with planning. My mother told me many years ago, I am the sort of woman who 'gets on with it' and because I do that I won't get any help. I've heard about women having problems going to back to work, because things have changed. And by gum they have changed. I heard one acquaintance of mine speaking about a work colleague who had returned to work and was off again after a short while. The acquaintance said, 'I think she was just wanting attention, sympathy, the whole thing's behind her now.' Have some patience, a lot has changed for that woman.

I know I'm lucky because I refused any further treatment, so I didn't have to experience 'that' (further treatment), each and everyone of us have our own 'that', and I believe, yes that made things easier for me. But it was a major operation. Six months down the line, I'm frustrated by the lack of strength in my left arm and around my shoulder (and my Pilates teacher Sara says it's to be expected!). Yes I look fine, there are things I can't do – carry heavy shopping, wield grandchildren about, carry my suitcase down the stairs. It's all tiring and I have to be careful in case I pull something again ☺

Anyway, the point of this chapter is: as long as I was 'off sick' I received some money and that was okay; but I am self-employed, I have a business and there was something strange happening in 2009 in respect of the 'recession', the 'credit crunch', whatever that was. (I did notice none of this seemed to stop lots of people spending like mad on the latest consumer must-have bargain, not always a bargain if you look closely at the quality of some of things). Lots of these purchases were about 'making people feel good'.

NLP note here: the only person that can make you feel good is you. You are response-able. Able to respond, the only person who takes full responsibility for you. Ok, sometimes we have to put ourselves in someone else's hands (like in the operating theatre). However, you're the one who can make decisions, who can argue your point and get want you want for you.

Anyway during this 'recession', I decided I needed to get my business back on track, on the road again. I'd been missing for around 4 months from the business scene. In fact one of clients asked me 'where the bloody hell have you been?' I told him. 'Oh,' he said, 'but you're all right now?' And yes I felt I was.

As I mentioned previously, some people, colleagues, business people, friends had made decisions on my behalf. Decisions about how I was, how I should be. Even 6 months down the line. I meet people who look at me and say 'but you look so well.' In my mind I ask 'how on earth do you expect me to look?' I do say that I didn't have any treatment, I'm sparkling with thoughts of what I want to achieve (the getting thinner is not going so well, exercise will have to be carried out – by me) and I'm thinking about what I want to avoid. Things to avoid are a useful part of Positive Thinking.

Planning: that's what I started out with.

My experience is that it would be really useful – for the self-employed, but also for the person on their own or the person on a low income (probably anyone really), to be given advice and/or a plan before they have the op. A week or so extra, unless you have some really rampant form of cancer, would

160

save you a lot of hassle when you come out and when your mind is feeling very well, your body is perhaps not so willing and you are getting mixed reactions from other people and if you are self-employed you are really wanting to get on with work.

I can't speak for others but I suspect there are plenty of women out there who would really like to know what happens afterwards, or what could happen. What steps can I take before I go into hospital? We need some patient care and prevention. The model seems to be – Cancer – do something about it (and yes great) – use big words and assume the patient has no idea what you are talking, that they don't want to know, on occasion talk about the patient as if she isn't there – assume everything will be a struggle, a fight, difficult, something to overcome – don't say too much as you need to cover your back in case the patient sues you later – and then 'let's fire fight'!

Planning, explaining, saves fire fighting. I agree there will be people who don't want to know, who will accept what they are told and give someone else the responsibility for their care, their life and then just blame others.

A plan, however, would save so many problems – this is what will happen – you will have this op – you will be in hospital for . . . days – when you get home, this is what you can do, this is who will visit you or not, this is what the hospital is responsible for, this is what your GP is responsible for, these are other places. (Oh yes, the JobCentre, and insurance company and anyone who deals with people who have had an op or who are in receipt of benefit, need to know what a mastectomy or a wide excision is. I prefer to tell people I've had a mastectomy – because 'cancer' usually sends their brains elsewhere – 'major surgery' means nothing, but there are many people who don't know what a mastectomy means. In one organisation out of three different women I spoke to only one knew what a mastectomy is! Education please!)

And then in respect of the plan, each woman and her family or significant needs a plan beforehand, so that when she goes back to work she can really go back to work and get on with her life.

NLP stuff: A possible way to plan

Answer all of the questions below. Get someone else to read these out to you preferably and to write your answers; you can think better that way. If some of the questions don't make sense, then go onto the next question, just leave that oneout. When you've finished, then sit together and start to work out what you could do and where you need to go to ask more questions.

When all of your treatment is finished, how and where do you want to be when you go back to work, to your family?

What are you going/working towards?

Where and how and from whom will you get support when you go back to work, 'get things back to normal'?

What will this support look like?

What will this support sound like?

What will this support feel like?

How will you feel?

Are you able to ask for this support?

What sequence of steps or stages will you need to put in place to achieve what you want?

What will this help you to avoid?

How will you divide what you want into small enough chunks or steps so that each one is do-able?

What else needs to be there for you to achieve this and for you to know that this will really support you?

Is what you want right for you in all circumstances in your life?

Is what you want appropriate for your personal relationships?

What will it give you that you might not have had, after your op?

What will having this plan cause you to lose?

Does any part of you object to putting all of this in place?

(If so how will you deal with that?)

Is it within your power or ability to achieve this?

What is the first step?

Can you take this first step?

Are you able to deal with whatever happens during this process?

Where do you want this plan to be carried out?

When do you want this plan to be carried out?

How do you want this plan to be carried out?

And with whom do you want to carry out this plan?

What resources will you need? (This could be money, could be physical things, could be new skills, could be self-esteem/confidence.)

Who will you have to become?

Who else has achieved this outcome?

Have you ever done this before?

Do you know anyone who has?

How will you know when your plan is in place?

What will let you know that you have achieved this plan and that it's ready to implement?

Are there any adjustments you would like to make to make this even better?

Then make a written plan. And go ask questions. And see the 'Ten Top Tips to Survive the Healthcare System' (on the next page): they might be Canadian, but they will be useful anywhere.

NLP stuff: Ten Top Tips to Survive the Healthcare System

These ten top tips were written by Shelle Rose Charvet. Shelle is Canadian and author of *Words That Change Minds* and co-creator with Roger Bailey of the Language and Behaviour (LAB) Profile. I have been privileged to train with Shelle twice and am now a Trainer and Consultant of the LAB Profile.

1. Always assume that you have fallen through the cracks, unless you get proof to the contrary. No news is not good news. It may mean that someone forgot to do something. Medical care can be complicated and need a lot of co-ordination among large numbers of people.

2. Never blame anyone. Recognize that everyone working in the system is very busy and probably stressed-out. While you are only concerned with yourself, they are juggling dozens of people, or hundreds.

3. Create positive relationships with everyone who can help you. Introduce yourself to every nurse, receptionist, technician and doctor that you will need to see again. Ask them for their first name. Remember it or record it for quick reference.

Next time you see them establish rapport by using their first name and engaging them in personal chat before you get down to business. It only takes a few seconds. This will help ensure that you become more than just a file, and will give you some insight into what each person does. It also makes it easier to request things when you need to.

4. Apologize before you make a request. 'I'm sorry to bother you when you are so busy, but since I hadn't heard from you, I thought I'd better check whether you were able to make the appointment.' Canadians [and the British] naturally apologize for anything, even when we are not responsible. It's time we learned to use the power of apology. If you say you're sorry, you can ask for just about anything – and still be perceived as nice.

5. Take someone with you and give them a job to do. For any important meeting or procedure, take a friend or family member with you. Their job is to remain sane, create rapport and ask good questions. This way, if you lose your grip, someone else still has it.

6. Use all your contacts. Surely someone you know, knows someone who knows someone who can find out what you need. At times this may be the only way to obtain information, a second opinion or to get in to see someone quickly. If you are hesitant to use your contacts, apologize for bothering them.

7. Be prepared to do a lot of waiting. Make appointments early in the day before the doctor has a chance to get behind schedule. This way you'll see the doctor before she/he gets tired and cranky. Just after lunch is okay too. Remember to take something you like to do in case you have to wait anyway.

8. Take everything your doctors say as information instead of gospel. Allow yourself time to think about it. Remember that medical professionals are trained to think about and discuss the worst possible scenarios. Ask them what each treatment is supposed to accomplish and repeat that message over and over to yourself to create a goal-oriented mindset within yourself. Write down your questions prior to the appointment and write down the answers – or ask your companion to do the writing.

9. Do what you need to do to stay upbeat and positive. It's perfectly normal to feel depressed and demoralized upon hearing bad news. I've been through shock, numbness, denying that this could be happening, panic, anger and feeling depressed. You can let yourself feel all those things, knowing that this is how you are feeling [sic] at this moment in time, and that you will move on. Continually remind yourself that you are good at healing, that you get better quickly. Notice what has improved each day and comment on it to yourself and others. While some may think this weird; you can even speak to your physical self; cheer for your immune system and thank it for sticking up for you.

10. Hang out with cheerful, upbeat and helpful people. I found it wearing having to cheer up other people when I told them I had cancer. I was also subjected to everyone's personal dogma regarding what I should do. It ran the gamut; from slavishly following every instruction from the doctor to never believing anything the doctor says. There is only so much sympathy you can take before you begin to believe that you ought to feel sorry for yourself. Only see people who make you feel good – who make you laugh, who get you out, who bring over lovely things to eat. If someone asks you how can they help – get them to make morale-raising food, take you to a funny movie, or bring over a good video. If depressing people want to come over, apologise and tell them you're not up to it.

Things I wish I'd known

1. You can pin the softee in your bra or top with a safety pin.

2. Massage your scar as soon as you get home after having the plaster off, in the morning and evening. No medical person told me this, this info came first from someone who had had a different op and later (much later) via other people, and only at my second appointment months later was I asked 'what are you massaging the scar with?' I used Weleda Rose Oil and later Golden Calendula Oil from Aromantics. I also used Bio Oil at one point and some, very expensive and not always reliable in terms of adhesive properties, scar-reducing plasters, but I worried about some of the contents of these products. I like the natural oils much better.

3. Everyone has the right to the services of a Macmillan nurse; I only discovered that over a year later. In the experiences we had with Michael, we had a Macmillan nurse, who was great with hints and tips guiding us in the right direction. I (wrongly) assumed you had to have terminal cancer or be undergoing some of kind of treatment. No one asked me, told me or pointed me in that direction this time.

Other women's stories

I decided I wanted to include some stories from other women in here, so that this book isn't just about 'that Rosie O'Hara, it's alright for her'. Getting stories was a challenge – for many reasons – here are some.

D's story

D was on the same ward as me. We have met a couple of times since then and she was happy to talk to me, but faded away a little when I mentioned I would like to publish her story, so I am allowed to say this.

She felt that as we are in Forres (NHS Grampian) and our operations were carried out in Inverness (NHS Highland) that we were rather left out. Like me, there were many things she didn't know, no physio follow-up. For her, being without a car meant that access to anywhere apart from where we live is fraught with difficulty: we are in a small town in the north-east of Scotland and buses are infrequent and expensive. There was no joined-up thinking in respect of patient care.

Richard's mum's story

Richard is a friend of mine; he's in his thirties, his mum slightly older than me. She had her mastectomy in York shortly before moving to Scotland; she had a horrendous experience, trust me we have much better care up here. The day she went into hospital she was told there was no bed for her! The op would go ahead; she had to wait in a corridor in front of the lifts and to walk to the operating theatre in her gown open at the back (this is in around 2006!). There was still no bed after her op, she was put in a general surgical ward. In the evening she felt lonely and worried, and she cried, the nurse on the ward eventually told her to 'shut up', that she couldn't help her because she knew nothing about mastectomies and that she was to stop being a baby! In the time she was in hospital, she never saw her surgeon and discharged herself on day 3 because she felt so upset and lonely. Within a week she moved to Scotland, I just cannot imagine that!

She had better care at Dr Gray's hospital in Elgin. She refused any further treatment as she already had existing health issues and didn't want her existing medication to conflict with any other. She was the one who told me about Macmillan nurses.

Sue's story

Sue sings in the same choir as I do, she had a wide excision and very kindly gave me her breast cancer diary. Thanks for sharing Sue ☺

'I was diagnosed with a grade 2 invasive carcinoma on 21st January 2009 in my left breast. The initial mammogram was done by the Highland Breast Screening Mobile Unit parked up in Tesco's car park. Being over 50, or 55 is it, years of age, I am eligible for regular breast screening. I did not have a lump but just some tissue which had become cancerous. It was nothing I could have felt by self-examination, I had no idea I had a problem. Anyway sure enough a letter followed shortly afterwards asking me to attend Raigmore Hospital for a further screening. Nothing to be alarmed about they said reassuringly in their letter as quite often anomalies turn up which need further investigation. The 19th January 2009 loomed and off I went to the hospital. Surprisingly there were three other ladies I knew from the village also there so they must have had a high take-up for the screening in Forres this year. I had a further mammogram, and ultrasound and a core biopsy. They were very thorough and extremely friendly. After all the procedures I had a talk with a breast care nurse who was able to tell me that I had one of the most common breast cancers (good to know I'm common)! The nurse was able to tell me that after the operation to remove the tissue which would probably be day surgery my treatment would probably consist of a course of twenty radiotherapy treatments and hormone tablets for 5 years. I would have to wait a couple of days for the results of the core biopsy and they said they would ring me on the Wednesday (21st January) after 17.00 p.m.

'Sure enough the telephone call arrived. I was at home on my own as my husband was working abroad and our two daughters live away.

The result was they had found some cancer cells during the core biopsy which had started to become invasive in the infected tissue. This would mean an overnight stay in hospital to see if the cancer had spread to my lymph nodes in my armpit. It was not easy hearing this news and I thought how do I tell my girls. Nobody in my family to my knowledge had ever had a cancer of any sort. I was just one of the unlucky ones (one in every 2,000 or so)! My husband suggested I told my oldest sister first to practice how I was to tell the girls which was a good idea. My sister is eleven years older than me and of a Christian persuasion so it was good to speak to her. When I did pluck up courage and speak to my girls later that night I told them it was a very common cancer and a small one (1.3 cm) and not hereditary so they should not worry. I rang the Breast Cancer Care Support Line the next day and spoke to a lovely lady who talked me through everything and reassured me. An appointment had been made for me to see the surgeon on 25th January so my elder daughter rang me back later that evening to say that she, her husband and daughter would come up on the Friday. Her husband and daughter would stay overnight and she would catch the train back on the Tuesday and accompany me to the hospital on the Monday. I had arranged to go out for a meal on that Friday night with a keep fit class so she said 'carry on and go and we will pick up a take away'. Life has to go on, so I did. We did not break down in tears when she arrived. I was worried that if I went to pieces so would she, so we kept it together. Her husband and daughter went back the next day but we had a lovely four days together, just the two of us, enabling us to do a bit of mother and daughter bonding. She had also had a brush with breast cancer a few weeks earlier but didn't want to tell me until she was sure everything was fine, which it was in her case. So when there was nothing to worry about, she told me, which was how I treated my problem as I did not tell anyone in the family about my second mammogram except my husband.

'The 25th January, the day of the visit to surgeon: my daughter took a pen and paper just in case we forgot to ask any particular questions and for her to write down the surgeon's comments so I wouldn't forget what was said. The operation would be done within 3 weeks and I could expect to be in overnight. It was to be a wide excision lumpectomy with a number of lymph nodes removed from my armpit for checking. It was hoped I would have radiotherapy and hormone tablets as my follow-up treatment. The surgeon showed us the mammograms so we could see the problem area. I did get a letter saying the date of the operation had been brought forward to 5th February. Why was it brought forward, was there some urgency that I hadn't been made aware of? No you are just panicking, half-term was the following week and the surgeon was trying to re-arrange his operating list to accommodate his patients, phew! On Monday 2nd February I had an appointment with my own GP for the results of a blood test as I have been on the verge of type 2 diabetes for a couple of years now. This confirmed that yes my blood sugar was high, and my liver had ten times as much of something (I can't remember what it was) that a healthy liver should have and whilst I was in having the breast operation he would arrange for me to have a liver scan done too! Of course I panicked again, don't tell me they have found cancer in my liver as well and now I'm diabetic. When I got home from the doctors I just broke down – as if I didn't have enough to cope with. By now my husband had left his job abroad and was home. I was back at the doctors the next day to get some tranquillisers to try and settle myself before going into hospital, which helped.

'The day of the operation was 5th February and I was schedule for the afternoon list. It was a wintry, snowy day and we arrived at Raigmore for checking in at 8.00 a.m. My husband left about an hour later after I had had all my paperwork checked. Lunch smelt really nice on the ward but I wasn't allowed any because of the afternoon operation. All I'd had since 20.00 p.m. the night before was a cup of tea that morning. It was the next day before I was properly out of the anaesthetic and I felt fine just a bit tender. I couldn't have breakfast or lunch that day because of having the liver scan in the afternoon (I was ravenous). The scan showed I had a couple of gallstones: what a relief that was! I was so worried that things were really going to be serious. Breast cancer, gallstones, diabetes all in 1 week, give me a break!

'Next appointment is the post-op one with the surgeon. The operation had gone well and they removed all the cancerous tissue in my breast an area of about two and a half inches just to be sure he had taken all the infected tissue and the five lymph nodes from my armpit closest to the infected tissue in my breast. Unfortunately one of the lymph nodes tested positive for cancer so it will mean treating that area with radiotherapy as well. There is no further need for surgery but I will now need to see the breast oncologist to get the radiotherapy treatment set up. There was a waiting list of about 8 weeks before treatment can start! I thought it would all be done by Easter but now it is not even likely to start before Easter!

'On Wednesday 18th March, my husband and I had a meeting with the breast oncologist to discuss the best form of treatment, the dreaded chemotherapy or radiotherapy. In my case, I was not going to gain a great deal more success with chemotherapy so it was decided to go with the surgeon's recommendation of radiotherapy and hormone tablets. The oncologist said she wanted to do a four-field therapy to make the treatment more accurate. The treatment is due to start on 18th May but starting on 18th March I will be taking Arimidex which is an anti-cancer drug for my particular type of breast cancer (HER2, I think).

'Thursday 25th April, I was at Raigmore Hospital to attend the planning treatment session. This is so they can set up the machine for my radiotherapy which will take about an hour or longer to get the precise co-ordinates downloaded for my treatment. This included more x-rays and tattoos which are the size of a full stop to make sure the treatment is guided to the correct area. The measurements are taken using something like a compass with curves at the end to encompass a breast and they put pink felt pen marks around my breast and used some kind of sticky markers which they removed after each picture. The camera and technology they used on Thursday wouldn't clear the top of my lung for treatment so I went back the following Wednesday to have a CT [computed tomography] scan done which will give a 3-D image and make the co-ordinates more accurate, allowing them to bend the beam so that less of my lung is compromised in the treatment. The four-field treatment means targeting the lymph glands in the top of my shoulder/lower neck, armpit, the breast on the site where the cancer was located and a place to the right of my breast closer to the breast bone. This means my whole breast will be irradiated. I will have to go back a couple of weeks later so that they can be sure that the first measurements will match up with the CT scan.

'The twenty treatments started on 18th May. Piece of doddle. I have been catching the bus as I have a bus pass and if I do feel tired I don't have to bother about the driving, traffic, parking, etc. What a fabulous team of radiotherapists they have there. All very nice and making you laugh and telling you what you could expect as the treatment progressed. I didn't feel particularly tired, but I did get a sore nipple towards the end (breastfeeding pads from the chemist with the moisturising cream on did the trick), and I did get a sensation of trying to swallow a golf ball towards the end of the course but everything felt fine. All a bit of a nuisance really more than anything. I have not felt ill at all and have just carried on as normal.

'17th June, last treatment session. They told me I still have 2 weeks worth of radiotherapy stored inside me so if I have an side effects they will last a couple of weeks yet.

'In January I thought I had been handed a death sentence but I can honestly say that I have not felt any ill effects whatsoever (bearing in mind I did not have chemotherapy which is entirely different) and sometimes felt a fraud as I kept asking the staff 'when am I going to feel ill'. Once the final 2 weeks is up, my red blood cells should return to normal and any side effects easing off.

'I had a check-up with the surgeon to make sure I was recovering well a few months later. He cannot say I am cured as there is no cure as yet. I asked him about the possibility of having an MRI [magnetic resonance imaging] scan to just to check that the cancer hadn't travelled any further and he said it would cost between £600–800 and could throw up any amount of non-life threatening diagnoses which would give me more to worry about. His advice – haven't you got anything else you would rather spend the money on – just MOVE ON! That's easy for him to say but it's my peace of mind I'm looking at. I didn't have the MRI scan and I am slowly moving on! This treatment has hopefully mopped up any stray cells and I hope to stay clear for the next 5 years. I will be examined every year now instead of every three. Apart from a scar on my left breast and under my left armpit, that is all there is and they have faded very well now, but I do have a dimple on the edge of my left breast.

'There will always be a 'what if' in my life now and it is the 'moving on' part I have had most difficulty with. Every time I get an ache, pain, twinge, I find myself saying 'Oh no, what if' and this has given rise to anxiety and panic attacks but I am gradually managing to conquer these fears with medication from my GP.

'During this past year I have met so many ladies in my own village who have had breasts removed, undergone chemo, some had no treatment at all; I was beginning to think I was joining the Amazon tribe. The tribe of women who hacked off their left breast so they could carry their shield and fight! What a wonderful support they have all been, offering lifts if need be and just generally taking the time to ask 'How are you today?'

'For anyone of breast-screening age, don't ignore the invitation to have the screening done. It was only the screening that found my problem as it was not anything I could feel.

'It makes you realise that you can no longer put things on hold you have to go out and seize the day whilst you still can.'

Jackie's story

Jackie very kindly agreed to meet with me and talk about her experiences. Thanks for sharing Jackie!

Jackie was diagnosed with breast cancer in May 2008, she had had incidences of fibrositis (cysts) and assumed it was another cyst, but after tests, the doctor she saw at the hospital said no, this was something serious and more tests would need to be done. Impressively, the doctors arranged to perform additional tests on the day! This included the first biopsy, when the doctor hit a vein. With the jolt of needle gun and the blood flowing from the vein. Jackie's friend Kirsty who was with her said 'it looked as she had been shot!' This was the first time the 'C' word was mentioned and the doctor gave a lovely description of the cancer being like a tree and the tests were to determine the variety of tree or type of cancer!

Jackie did lots of research on the internet and Kirsty's partner bought her books, including *Breast Cancer for Dummies*! Initial concerns about being left without a nipple diminished further into treatment.

Jackie went for several further appointments in Aberdeen and throughout the whole range of investigations, Jackie and Kirsty maintained a good level of hilarity, surprising some of the doctors and nursing staff.

Her operation eventually took place in August and she had a lumpectomy in which the lump was removed and breast tissue moved round so that her breast retained its shape. Prior to the operation, radioactive dye was injected into the nipple so the main lymph nodes could be identified and removed. This also produced a glorious blue pee the following day. The new breast looked very good but having the stitch removed from her nipple 10 days later was not one of her favourite things. Tests showed cancer was present in the tissues surrounding the lump and two of three lymph nodes were also cancerous so Jackie was informed she would need mastectomy and chemotherapy. Jackie opted for reconstruction at the time of the same time as the mastectomy.

She subsequently had the mastectomy and then, in the December, a tram-flap reconstruction – this means that tissue is taken from the stomach and the breast reconstructed using this tissue. It's a 12 hour operation, long enough for the surgeon to need a break to grab a sandwich.

After the reconstruction, she tells me she was 'cooked' for 2 days – that is, kept in a room on her own and at a high temperature (at this point in her life, her body, of course, decided it was time to start having hot flushes). This 'cooking' is to help the body accept the stomach tissue, and the 'flap' as the new breast is referred to is checked every 15 minutes to begin with for 24 hours to make sure the body is accepting the tissue.

The op went well and Jackie started chemotherapy at her local hospital, the first session was a doddle (or so she thought), no problems, drove self there and back, had something eat but was sick later. This resulted in her anti-nausea drugs being upped for the next round. For the last three rounds, she had to travel to Aberdeen (one and a half hours away) as she needed a special cocktail of chemo drugs. (Travelling there nowadays means a trip to Sainsbury's – we don't have one locally).

When her hair fell out, Jackie got a blonde bob wig on the NHS. Her hair didn't 'fall out in handfuls' as people had told her, she says, but she was waiting for and wanting it to fall out as, to her, that was the indication the chemo was working. But the wig was too hot (along with the hot flushes) and she turned to bandanas. Everyone who came to the house had to be photographed wearing the wig.

Now she has been taken Tamoxifen but this will change to Arimidex and she goes for her mammograms regularly. Her remaining real breast has a mammogram, not the reconstruction as that is different tissue (in the USA there is a Trammogram!).

NLP stuff: On getting other people to 'go with you'

Or in the words of Shelle Rose Charvet,[22] 'meeting the person at their bus stop and getting them to come with you'.

1. With hindsight I realise that on 26th January 2009 when I really needed Jim on my side, I will have used phrases like 'we need to prevent things from getting worse', 'help me get rid of these problems', 'I can't do this on my own', 'this is how I want to fix it so that it won't deteriorate' and 'I refuse to deal with this again, so I'm changing my diet, I'm avoiding negative people and what they have to say'.

2. In my head I was saying to me 'the positive consequences of this will be . . .', 'the advantages of this way of speaking are [I'll get him on my side by speaking about avoiding problems]', 'I'm interested in the benefits for me and Jim' and 'my goal is to have something to look forward to and get that, my compelling purpose, being with Jim, being with my grandsons and being there for their Mum'.

---

[22] Shelle has written two books, *Words That Change Minds* and *The Customer is Bothering Me*, both using the Language and Behaviour Profile . The former has been by my side and in my training and daily life for many years. As a trainer and consultant of the LAB Profile, I have really walked my talk many times with this form of language use.

To me, problems, mountains, obstacles are there to be got round or I want to make a hole in wall, build a door and get through things, so the language in the first paragraph is not mine in respect of getting well, in some contexts, I do think about what I want to avoid, not this one ☺ Apart from staying in hospital for too long.

3. I also asked Jim to think it through and understand the situation from my point of view (asking him to listen was inappropriate at this point – I needed him to see clearly something he can do and I needed to get him out of his feelings and to look up and see our future). He needed to consider.

4. When all I wanted to do was just go for it, jump in, now, get it done, make it happen.

5. I said I knew there was very much a right way for the medical profession, that it was tried and tested, and that there was a process and a step by step, but this was about me

6. And I wanted other alternatives, there might have been something else useful, and I wanted to look at the possibilities.

And because I matched Jim's language patterns first and then gave him mine, in a very short space of time, he supported me and he still does. Even this morning, as I was leaving the house to go to my Pilates class (on time for once) and he asked me to do something for him and I begrudgingly did it for him (because as he said I can do it better than he can) and I told him I was annoyed (I hate being late for other people and I hate it when others do that to me in a training session and I was annoyed at me), Jim said with a twinkle in his eyes 'yes well we have wordies and then it's alright isn't it?' Strong stuff this language.

In the LAB Profile, the language in the paragraph 1 is Away From, in 2 it's Towards. Paragraph 3 is Reactive language and 4 is Proactive, whereas 5 is about Procedures and 6 is about Options. My rule of thumb for identifying another person's language patterns is – whatever language or reaction is painful for you (when said or carried about by another person), this is someone using the opposite of the language you use. Meet them at their bus stop and they'll come with you and life will be easier (trust me on this one).

And I almost forgot to say

Eventually a year, well a little more than a year, after my op I went back for a further mammogram, I wondered how you carry out a mammogram of the non-existent breast and when I asked the radiographer – these women are lovely I tell you, yah boo sucks to all the in-my-opinion daft comments and jokes about mammograms – I said to her 'I'm really perplexed about how you do this, there's no boob there.' She simply looked at me and said, 'Ah yes. It's stupid isn't it, no one tells you it's the one that's left that we take a mammogram of.' 'Doh,' I thought. She said, 'a valid question.'

Anyway, after that and some faffing over three questions I had, which the doctor I saw couldn't answer and had to fetch my surgeon in, who was in a hurry as he was trying to fit three clinics into 1 week, as it was now the school holidays and note Sue's diary (we have the same surgeon) he takes school holidays off, so does his wife and she's one of the breast care nurses! My surgeon looked at me and rolled his eyes and said 'oh, you would have questions' in a nice tonality. I had two thoughts, one 'well that's your model of the world and you are rushing' and the other 'well, pay attention when it's me and save yourself the trouble and see me yourself, I will always be asking questions and I've saved the NHS a fortune, no radiotherapy, no medication!'

It's working for me. My letter from him telling me I have an all clear is blue-tacked to a picture in our kitchen!

Out of alignment

In November 2010 something bizarre happened, which in part goes to show you never, ever stop learning. I went down to North Shields to take part in a course, some learning for me on coaching and mentoring for managers to help me with a problem I was having with one of our associates and me. The associate had already made their own decision prior to me actually getting to the course. Ah well. I went into the course with an open mind because it involved something called Clean Language. I'm never really sure whether I like this Clean Language or not, but apparently I use it, quite often!

Anyway on the first day we were asked to be what we are like when we are ready to learn. Now for some things, like many people around 'I can't or couldn't put that into words, I could show you'. So I showed the trainer Caitlin Walker that I had a feeling down the left side of my chest, as she came back to me questioned me a little further, I said something like 'I notice I need to move that feeling more to the centre of my body, as there's a bit missing'. Now I've known Caitlin for a lot of years and she smiled and nodded knowingly.

What is fascinating is that over the next 2 weeks I started to notice that I had been internally and subconsciously 'lopsided' for a while, probably about 1 year and almost 10 or 11 months. Well of course I've been doing all that concentrating on my left side and healing and I've gone off kilter. So as I write I'm still shifting my centred and grounded-ness to my centre (of my body) and noticing how my alert, learning state and healing state is there and that that's ok, I also have something like flu a this point in time and I'm hoping that all of this is a final way of getting rid of the all the rubbish.

Whatever you do or someone else chooses to do, it's your or their choice. Please support the person with the cancer in their choice.

Bibliography

Kaelin, Carolyn M. *The Breast Cancer Survivor's Fitness Plan*. McGraw Hill, 2007.

O'Connor, J and Seymour, J. *Introducing NLP*. Element, 1993.

O'Hara, Rosie. *Finding The Relationship You Deserve*. Penpress, 2008.

Rose Charvet, Shelle. *Words That Change Minds*. Kendal Hunt, 1995.

Weed, Susun S. *Breast Cancer? Breast Health! The Wise Woman Way*. Ash Tree Publishing, 1996.

Contact Rosie O'Hara through www.nlphighland.co.uk

Glossary of NLP terminology

Associated/association
Mentally seeing, hearing, and feeling from inside an experience. In contrast to **Dissociated** (seeing a representation from the outside, as a spectator).

Auditory (A)
Representational system of hearing. Can be internal or external.

Auditory digital (Ad)
Representational system dealing with logic and the way we talk to ourselves.

Calibration
The ability to notice and measure changes for a standard that is applicable to a person. This is usually the comparison between two different sets of external, non-verbal cues.

Dissociated	Stepping apart from, and out of, an experience, seeing or hearing watching yourself.
First Position	One of the **Perceptual Positions**. First Position is when you are **Associated**, looking through your own eyes, and in touch with your own inner **Model of the World**.
Gustatory (G)	**Representational system** dealing with taste.
Internal Representations	How we re-present information to ourselves this will include Pictures, Sounds, Feelings, Tastes and Self-Talk.
Kinesthetic (K)	**Representational system** in respect of feelings, tactile experiences.

Lead representational system	The **Representational system** used to access stored information and lead it from the Unconscious Mind to the Conscious Mind.
Limiting belief	Beliefs or decisions we make about ourselves and/or our model of the world that limit the way we live.
Limiting decision	The decision that preceded the adoption of a **Limiting belief.**
Meta	Something that it is at a higher level (often out of conscious awareness).
Meta Position	A fly on the wall position similar to **Third Position.**
Model of the World	A person's values, beliefs and attitudes as well as their internal representations, states and

physiology, that all relate to and create the person's belief system of how the world operates. Also known as Map of the World.

Neuro Linguistic Programming (NLP) The process of creating human excellence in which usefulness is the most important criteria for success. The study of the structure of subjective experience. It is a process developed by a group of individuals who wished to explore new perceptions of reality and gain practical methods for themselves and others to develop their thinking, well-being and success. NLP now embraces many ideas and 'tools' taken and adapted from many other disciplines. These tools are useful in self-development. The best practitioners of NLP are those who have the courage, openness and flexibility to develop themselves using all methods available to them.

Nominalisation A noun describing a state of being which exists in name only. It can be a verb or another process word that has been formed into an abstract noun and then 'frozen in time'.

Olfactory (O) Representational system dealing with smell.

Perceptual Position We know from our experience of everyday life, that not everyone shares our point of view; so in order to understand a situation fully it's useful to take on different perspectives, just as if you were viewing an object from different angles to get an idea of its width, height and length. So for example being in Second Position is about understanding things from the other person's point of view 'being in their shoes as them' and using some good listening skills.

Projection

To attribute your ideas or feelings to other people or to another **Model of the World**.

Rapport

The ability to relate to other people in a way that creates trust and understanding.

Reframing

Process of making a shift in the nature of a problem or changing the structure or context of a statement to give it another meaning.

Representational systems

The Sensory Modalities – **Visual**, **Auditory**, **Kinesthetic**, **Olfactory** and **Gustatory**. Called representational because it is the way in which memories and ideas are re-presented in our brains.

Resourceful State	The total experience when a person feels resourceful, confident and able to cope effectively
Second Position	In **Perceptual Positions**, Second Position is usually someone else's point of view.
Third Position	In **Perceptual Positions**, Third Position is a **Meta Position**, is the point of view of a dissociated observer (so you watching yourself), an overview.
Timeline	How you unconsciously arrange your past memories and future expectations. Typically seen as a 'line' of images.
Visual (V)	**Representational system** dealing with the sense of sight. It can be external or internal.

Also from MX Publishing

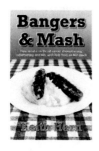

Bangers and Mash

Battling Throat Cancer with NLP
"Hern excellently describes living with cancer." The Lancet

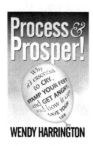

Process and Prosper

Eye opening book on surviving necrotizing faciitis.

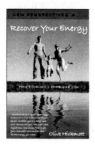

Recover Your Energy

NLP for Chronic Fatigue, ME and tiredness

More NLP books at www.mxpublishing.co.uk

Also From MX Publishing

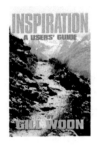

Inspiration, A Users Guide

A travel guide to inspiration full of hints and tips from an NLP practitioner.

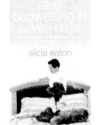

Stop Bedwetting in 7 Days

A simple step-by-step guide to help children conquer bedwetting problems in just a few days

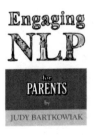

Engaging NLP for Parents

From a series of books covering practical tips from NLP. See also NLP for New Mums, NLP for Teens and several more.

More NLP books at www.mxpublishing.co.uk

Also from MX Publishing

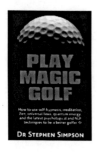

Play Magic Golf

How to use self-hypnosis, meditation, Zen, universal laws, quantum energy, and the latest psychological and NLP techniques to be a better golfer

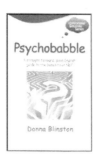

Psychobabble

A straight forward, plain English guide to the benefits of NLP

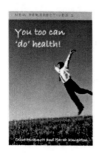

You Too Can Do Health

Improve Your Health and Wellbeing, Through the Inspiration of One Person's Journey of Self-development and Self-awareness Using NLP, energy and the Secret Law of Attraction

More NLP books at www.mxpublishing.co.uk